THE POWER OF THE VAGUS NERVE

ACTIVATE THE VAGUS NERVE WITH SELF-HELP EXERCISE FOR DEPRESSION, ANXIETY, TRAUMA AND CHRONIC INFLAMMATION.

AUTHOR:

ETHELINE BOUVIER

CONTENTS

PART TWO

INTRODUCTION

The vagus nerve is made of a long bundle of sensory and motor fibers that link the brainstem to the chest, lungs, and intestines. It also branches to the liver, spleen, gallbladder, ureter, female reproductive organs, head, tongue, and kidneys to contact and communicate. This feeds our subconscious nervous center, the parasympathetic nervous system, which regulates the body's unconscious functions, as well as everything from maintaining our heart rate and digestion to breathing and sweating steadily. It also asssits to regulate blood pressure and to balance blood glucose, encourages general renal function, helps release bile and testosterone, induces saliva production, helps control taste, triggers tears, and plays a major role in fertility and women's orgasms.

Vagus nerve dysfunction can cause a lot of problems that include obesity, bradycardia (abnormally slow heart rate), difficulty swallowing, gastrointestinal diseases, fainting, mood disorders, vitamin B12 deficiency, chronic inflammation, impaired cough and seizures.

Meanwhile, it has been shown that vagus nerve stimulation improves conditions such as:

- Poor blood circulation
- Mood disorder
- Cancer

- Anxiety disorder
- Heart disease
- Tinnitus
- Leaky intestine
- Poor blood circulation
- Mood disorder
- Cancer
- Obesity
- Alcohol addiction
- Migraines
- Alzheimer's

A CLOSER LOOK AT THIS SUPER NERVE

The vagus nerve is the longest of our 12 cranial nerves. Only the spine is a larger nervous system. About 80% of its nerve fibers, or four of its five "tracks", carry information from the body to the brain. Its fifth path goes in the opposite direction, sending signals from the brain to the whole body. Anchored in the brainstem, the base spreads from the neck to the chest and divides into two, left and right. Each of these pathways is made up of tens of thousands of nerve fibers that branch into the heart, lungs, stomach, pancreas, and almost every other organ in the abdomen.

The vagus nerve uses acetylcholine, a neurotransmitter, which stimulates muscle contractions in the parasympathetic nervous system. A neurotransmitter is a type of chemical messenger released at the end of a nerve fiber, which allows signals to pass from one point to another, stimulating multiple organs. For example, if our brain could not communicate with our diaphragm by releasing acetylcholine through the vagus nerve, we would stop breathing.

Vagus nerve lesions can be caused by diabetes, alcoholism, viral infections of the upper respiratory tract or accidental rupture of part of the nerve during an operation. Stress can ignite the nerve, as well as fatigue and anxiety. Even something as simple as bad posture can negatively affect the vagus nerve.

CHAPTER 1

THE POLYVAGAL THEORY

The polyvagal theory describes an autonomous nervous system that is influenced by the central nervous system, sensitive to afferent influences, characterized by an adaptive reactivity dependent on the phylogeny of neuronal circuits, and interactive with the source nuclei in the brainstem that regulates the striated muscles of the face and head. The theory depends on the accumulated knowledge that describes the phylogenetic transitions in the autonomic nervous system of vertebrates. Its specific focus is on the phylogenetic change between reptiles and mammals that resulted in specific changes in the vagal pathways that regulate the heart. As the nuclei of the primary vagal efferent pathways that regulate the heart changed from the dorsal motor nucleus of the vagus in reptiles to the ambiguous nucleus in mammals, a face-heart connection evolved with the emerging properties of a social engagement system that would allow social interactions to regulate visceral state.

The regulation of the central nervous system of visceral organs is the focus of several historical publications that have shaped the texture of physiological research. For example, in 1872 Darwin recognized the dynamic neuronal relationship between the heart and the brain:

"when the heart is affected, it reacts in the brain; and the state of the brain reacts again through the pneumogastric [vagus] nerve in the heart; so that, under any emotion, there is a lot of mutual action and reaction between these, the two most important organs of the body..."

Although Darwin recognized the two-way communication between the viscera and the brain, the subsequent formal description of the autonomic nervous system has minimized the importance of central and afferent regulatory structures. After Langley, medical and physiological research tended to focus on the peripheral motor nerves of the autonomic nervous system, with a conceptual emphasis on matched antagonism between the sympathetic and parasympathetic efferent pathways in the target visceral organs. This approach has minimized interest in both afferent pathways and in brain stem areas that regulate specific efferent pathways.

The early conceptualization of the idea focused on an efferent undifferentiated path that would have to modulate the "tone" simultaneously with different target organs. Therefore, the areas of the brainstem that regulate the supra-diaphragmatic (e.g. Myelinated vaginal pathways that originate in the ambiguous nucleus and extend mainly above the diaphragm) were not functionally distinct from those that regulate the diaphragm (e.g. Non-myelinated vagal pathways originating in the dorsal motor nucleus of the vagus and ending mainly under the diaphragm).Without this contrast, research and theory focused on the antagonism coupled between parasympathetic and sympathetic innervation to the target organs. The consequence of an emphasis on matched antagonism was the acceptance in physiology and medicine of global constructions such as autonomous sympathetic tone and vagal tone balance.

Over 50 years ago, Hess proposed that the autonomic nervous system was not only vegetative and automatic, but that it was an integrated system with peripheral and central neurons. Underlining the central mechanisms that mediate the dynamic regulation of the peripheral organs, Hess anticipated the need for technologies to continuously monitor the peripheral and central neural circuits involved in the regulation of visceral function.

THE POLYVAGAL THEORY: THREE PHYLOGENETIC RESPONSE SYSTEMS

The study of the phylogeny of the autonomic nervous system of vertebrates provides a response to the vagal paradox. Research in correlative neuroanatomy and neurophysiology has identified two branches of the vagus, with each branch supporting different adaptive functions and behavioral strategies. The vagal output to the heart from a branch manifests itself in respiratory sinus arrhythmia and the output from the other branch is manifested in bradycardia and perhaps the slowest rhythms in the variability of heart rate. Although slower rhythms are thought to have a sympathetic influence, they are blocked by atropine.

The polyvagal theory illustrates how each of the three phylogenetic stages in the development of the vertebrate autonomic nervous system is associated with a distinct autonomous subsystem that is maintained and expressed in mammals. These autonomous subsystems are phylogenetically ordered and linked to social communication (e.g. facial expression, vocalization, listening), mobilization (e.g. fight-flight behavior) and immobilization (e.g. pretending death, vasovagal syncope and behavioral arrest).

The social communication system (i.e. the social commitment system; see below) involves the myelinated vagus, which serves to promote calm behavioral states by inhibiting sympathetic influences to the heart and dampening the hypothalamic-pituitary-adrenal axis (HPA 16). The mobilization system depends on the functioning of the sympathetic nervous system. The most phylogenetically primitive component, the immobilization system, depends on the unmyelinated vagus, which is shared with most vertebrates. With the increase in neural complexity arising from phylogenetic development, the organism's physiological and affective repertoire is enchanced. The three circuits can be vizualized as dynamic, providing adaptive responses to safe, dangerous and potentially lethal contexts and events.

Only mammals have a myelinated vagus. Unlike the unmyelinated vagus, which originates in the dorsal motor nucleus of the vagus with pre- and postganglionic muscarinic receptors, the myelinated mammalian vagus originates in the ambiguous nucleus, preganglionic nicotinic receptors and postganglionic muscarinic receptors. The non-myelinated vagus is shared with other vertebrates, including reptiles, amphibians, teleosts and elasmobranchs.

We are now studying the possibility of extracting different features of the heart rate model to dynamically oversee both the vagal systems. Initial studies in the laboratory support this possibility. In these studies, we blocked nicotinic preganglionic receptors with hexamethonium and muscarinic receptors with atropine. The data was collected from the prairie vole, which has a very high environmental vagal tone. These preliminary data showed that, in different animals, nicotinic block selectively removes the respiratory sinus arrhythmia without damping the amplitude of the lower frequencies in heart rate variability. In contrast, blockade of muscarinic receptors with atropine removes both low and respiratory frequencies.

The three cycles are organized and respond to challenges in a phylogenetically determined hierarchy consistent with the Jacksonian dissolution principle. Jackson proposed that in the brain, the higher neural circuits (ie, phylogenetically more recent) inhibit the lower neural circuits (ie, phylogenetically older) and "when the higher ones are suddenly rendered functionless, the lower increase in activity."18 Although Jackson proposed to disband to explain changes in brain function due to damage and disease, the polyvagal theory proposes a similar phylogenetically ordered hierarchical model to describe the sequence of strategies for autonomous response to challenges.

Functionally, if the environment is perceived as safe, two important characteristics are expressed. First, the body state is efficiently regulated to promote growth and restoration (i.e. visceral homeostasis). This occurs through an increase in the influence of the myelinated vagal motor pathways of mammals on the cardiac pacemaker which slows the heart, inhibits the mechanisms of flight control of the sympathetic nervous system, dampens the HPA axis stress response system (e.g. Cortisol) and reduces inflammation by modulating immune reactions (e.g. cytokines). Secondly, through the process of evolution, the nuclei of the brainstem that regulate the myelinated vagus have integrated with the nuclei that regulate the muscles of the face and head. This connection translates into the bidirectional coupling between spontaneous behaviors of social commitment and bodily states. In particular, a system of integrated social involvement emerged in mammals when the neural regulation of visceral states that promote growth and restoration (through the myelinated vagus) was linked neuroanatomically and neurophysiologically to the neuronal regulation of the muscles that control the gaze, the facial expression, listening and prosody.

The human nervous system, quite similar to that of other mammals, has evolved not only to survive in safe environments, but also to promote survival in dangerous and potentially lethal contexts. To achieve this adaptive flexibility, the human nervous system has maintained two more primitive neuronal circuits to regulate defensive strategies (i.e. the fight-or-flight and death behaviors). It is crucial to note that social behavior, social communication and visceral homeostasis are incompatible with the neurophysiological states and behaviors promoted by the two neuronal circuits that support defense strategies. Therefore, through evolution, the human nervous system maintains three neural circuits, which are located in an organized phylogenetic hierarchy. In this hierarchy of adaptive responses, the most recent circuit is used first; if that circuit does not provide security, the older circuits are recruited sequentially.

The investigation on the phylogenesis of the regulation of the vertebrate heart has led to the extraction of four principles that provide a basis for the verification of hypotheses related to specific neural mechanisms of social involvement, fight for flight and pretending death behaviors:

There is a phylogenetic change in the management of the heart from endocrine transmission to unmyelinated nerves and lastly to the myelinated nerves.

There is a deepening of opposing neural mechanisms of excitation and inhibition to provide rapid regulation of gradual metabolic production.

A face-heart connection evolved when the nuclei of origin of the vagal tracts moved ventrally from the nucleus of the older dorsal motor to the ambiguus of the nucleus. This involved an anatomical and neurophysiological link between the neural regulation of the heart through the myelinated vagus and the special visceral efferent pathways that regulate the striated muscles of the face and head, forming an integrated social involvement system

With an increase in cortical development, the cortex shows greater control over the brainstem through direct neural pathways (e.g. corticobulbar) and indirect ones (e.g. corticoreticulars) that originate in the motor cortex and terminate in the nuclei of origin of the myelinated motor nerves that emerge also from the brain stem as somatomotor structures (muscles of the face and head).

NEUROCEPTION: CUEING CONTEXTUAL OF ADAPTIVE AND MALADAPTIVE PHYSIOLOGICAL STATES

To effectively pass from defensive strategies to those of social commitment, the mammalian nervous system must perform two important adaptive tasks: (1) assess the risk and (2) if the environment is perceived as safe, inhibit the most primitive limbic structures that they control the fight, flight or freezing behavior.

Any stimulus that has the potential to increase the safety experience of an organism has the potential to recruit the evolutionarily advanced neural circuits that hold the prosocial behaviors of the social engagement system.

The nervous system, through the handling of sensory information from the environment and from the viscera, constantly assesses the risk. Since the neural risk assessment does not require conscious awareness and may involve subcortical limbic structures, the term neuroception has been introduced to emphasize a neural process, distinct from perception, able to distinguish environmental (and visceral) characteristics that are safe, dangerous, or potentially lethal. In safe environments, the autonomous state is adaptively regulated to dampen sympathetic activation and protect the central nervous system dependent on oxygen, in particular the cortex, from the metabolically conservative reactions of the vagal dorsal complex. However, how does the nervous system determines when the environment is safe, dangerous or life-threatening and what neural mechanisms evaluate this risk?

ENVIRONMENTAL COMPONENTS OF NEUROCEPTION

Neuroception is a neural process that allows humans and other mammals to engage in social behavior by distinguishing safe contexts from dangerous contexts. Neuroception is proposed as a plausible mechanism that mediates both the expression and the interruption of positive social behavior, the regulation of emotions and visceral homeostasis. since the limbic reactivity is modulated by the responses of the temporal cortex to the intention of voices, faces and hand movements. Therefore, the neuroception of familiar individuals and individuals with adequately prosodic voices and warm and expressive faces translates into a social interaction that promotes a sense of security.

In most individuals (i.e. those without a psychiatric disorder or neuropathology), the nervous system assesses the risk and matches the neurophysiological status with the real risk of the environment. When the environment is assessed as safe, defensive limbic structures are inhibited, allowing for the social involvement and calmness of visceral states. On the contrary, some individuals experience a discrepancy and the nervous system evaluates the environment as dangerous even when it is safe. This discrepancy results in physiological states that support fighting, escape or freezing behaviors, but not social involvement behaviors. According to the theory, social communication can be efficiently expressed through the social engagement system only when these defensive circuits are inhibited.

OTHER CONTRIBUTORS TO NEUROCEPTION

Risk characteristics in the environment do not only drive neuroception. The afferent feedback from the viscera provides an important mediator of the accessibility of the prosocial circuits associated with social involvement behaviors. For example, the polyvagal theory predicts that states of mobilization would compromise our ability to detect positive social signals. Functionally, visceral states color our perception of objects and others. Therefore, the same characteristics of a person that involves another person can determine a series of results, depending on the physiological state of the target individual. If the person involved is in a state where the social commitment system is easily accessible, mutual prosocial interactions are likely to occur. However, if the individual is in a state of mobilization, one could respond to the same engaging response with the asocial characteristics of withdrawal or aggression. In such a state, it could be very difficult to dampen the mobilization circuit and allow the social commitment system to come back online.

The insula may be involved in mediating neuroception, as it has been proposed as a brain structure involved in transmitting diffuse feedback from viscera to cognitive awareness. Functional imaging experiments have shown that the insula plays an important role in the experience of pain and in the experience of different emotions, including anger, fear, disgust, happiness and sadness. Critchley proposes that internal body states are represented in the insula and contribute to subjective feeling states, and has shown that activity in the insula is correlated with interoceptive accuracy.

SUMMARY

The polyvagal theory adduces that the evolution of the autonomic nervous system of mammals provides the neurophysiological substrates for adaptive behavioral strategies. It also proposes that the physiological state limits the range of behaviors and psychological experience. The theory links the evolution of the autonomic nervous system to affective experience, emotional expression, facial gestures, voice communication and contingent social behavior. In this way, the theory provides a plausible explanation for the covariation reported between atypical autonomic regulation (e.g. reduced vagal and major heart influences) and psychiatric and behavioral disorders that lead to difficulties in regulating appropriate social, emotional and communicative behaviors.

Polyvagal theory provides different insights into the adaptive nature of the physiological state. First of all, the theory emphasizes that physiological states support different classes of behavior. For example, a physiological state characterized by a vagal withdrawal would support the fight and flight mobilization behaviors. On the contrary, a physiological state characterized by an increased vagal influence on the heart (through myelinated vagal pathways originating from the ambiguous nucleus) would support spontaneous behavior of social involvement. Secondly, the theory emphasizes the formation of a system of social involvement integrated through functional and structural connections between the neural control of striated muscles of the face and the smooth muscles of the viscera. Third, the polyvagal theory proposes a mechanism - neuroception - to trigger or inhibit defense strategies.

CHAPTER 2

AUTONOMIC NERVOUS SYSTEM

The autonomic nervous system oversees a variety of bodily processes that occur without conscious act. The autonomic system is the part of the peripheral nervous system responsible for regulating the involuntary functions of the body, such as heart rate, blood flow, digestion and respiration.

THE DESIGN OF THE AUTONOMIC NERVOUS SYSTEM

This system is further splited into three branches:

- the sympathetic system,
- the parasympathetic system,
- the enteric nervous system.

The sympathetic part of the autonomic nervous system regulates the escape or fight responses. This division also performs tasks such as relaxing the bladder, accelerating the heart rate and dilating the pupils.

The parasympathetic part of the autonomic nervous system helps maintain normal bodily functions and conserves physical resources. This division also performs tasks such as bladder control, narrowing of the pupils and slowing heart rate .

The autonomic nervous system also consists of a third factor known as the enteric nervous system, which is limited to the gastrointestinal tract.

The autonomic nervous system works by receiving information from the environment and from other areas of the body system. The parasympathetic and sympathetic systems tend to have opposite actions in which one system will stimulate a response in which the other will inhibit it.

Traditionally, it was thought that stimulation occurred through the sympathetic system while it was thought that inhibition occurred through the parasympathetic system. However, many exceptions have been found to this.

For example, the sympathetic nervous system will react to increase blood pressure while the parasympathetic nervous system will react to lower it. The two systems work together to manage the body's responses according to the situation and needs. If, for example, you are facing a risk and need to escape, the sympathetic system will quickly mobilize your body to act. Once the risk has passed, the parasympathetic system will then begin to dampen these responses, slowly bringing your body back to its normal resting state.

WHAT DOES THE AUTONOMIC NERVOUS SYSTEM DO?

The autonomic system controls a variety of internal processes including:

- Digestion
- Blood pressure
- Heart rate frequency
- Emotional responses
- Urination and defecation
- Metabolism
- Electrolyte balance
- Pupil response
- Respiratory rate (respiration)
- Sexual response
- Body temperature
- Production of body fluids including sweat and saliva

Autonomic nerve pathways connect different organs to the brainstem or spinal cord. There are also two major neurotransmitters, or chemical messengers, essential for communication inside the autonomic nervous system:

Acetylcholine is mostly used in the parasympathetic system to have an restraining effect.

Norepinephrine works within the sympathetic system to have a stimulating effect on the body.

PROBLEMS WITH THE AUTONOMIC NERVOUS SYSTEM

When the sympathetic and parasympathetic components of the autonomic nervous systems are not in sync, people will experience an autonomic disorder, referred to as dysautonomia.

There are different types of autonomic disorders, each with its own unique set of symptoms, including:

- Acute autonomic paralysis
- Affective failure of baroreflex
- Idiopathic orthostatic hypotension
- Atrophy of the multiple system
- Orthostatic hypotension
- Postprandial hypotension
- Pure autonomic failure
- Family dysautonomia (Riley-Day syndrome)
- Secondary orthostatic hypotension

These disorders can occur on their own or as a result of other conditions that cause disorders of the autonomic nervous system, including:

- Autoimmune disease
- Alcohol or drug abuse
- Diabetes
- Parkinson's disease
- Cancer
- Chronic fatigue syndrome
- Peripheral neuropathy
- Aging

- Spinal cord disorders
- Trauma

THE SYMPTOMS

If you or someone you love experience disorders of the autonomic nervous system, it is possible that one or more of the following symptoms may occur. Some people experience a group of symptoms simultaneously and another set of symptoms at other times. Symptoms can be momentary and unpredictable or triggered by specific situations or actions, such as after ingesting certain foods or getting up quickly.

- Dizziness or lightheadedness in an upright position
- Fatigue and inertia
- Erectile dysfunction
- Lack of sweat or heavy sweating
- Urinary incontinence
- Difficulty in emptying the bladder
- Lack of pupillary response
- Disturbing pains and aches
- Collapsing (or even real fainting spells)
- Tachycardia (fast heart rate)
- Hypotension (low blood pressure)
- Gastrointestinal symptoms
- Numbness and tingling
- Severe anxiety or depression

The autonomic nervous system plays a very essential role in the human body, controlling many of the body's automatic processes. This system also helps prepare the body for coping with stress and threats, as well as bringing the body back to a state of rest later. Learning more about this part of the nervous system can give you a better understanding of the processes that underlie many human behaviors and responses.

THE 12 CRANIAL NERVES

The 12 cranial nerves are the abdominal nerve, accessory, facial, glossopharyngeal, hypoglossal, oculomotor, olfactory, optical, trigeminal, trochlear, vagus and vestibule-cochlear. The functions of the cranial nerves are divided into the management of different aspects of your body's daily activities, from chewing and biting to motor function, hearing, smelling and vision.

Cranial nerve functions are sensory, motor or both:

Sensory cranial nerves help a person see, smell and feel.

Motor cranial nerves help control muscle movements of the head and neck.

The human brain possesses a number of different nerves that are distributed around the body, which serve to carry vital signals to and from the brain. The cranial nerves are twelve in all, but what are their respective functions?

The brain must have a complex system of nerves and connections with the rest of the body in order to control the various parts of the body. There are twelve different nerves that flow from the brain, out of the base of the skull and up to the various regions of the body. Most of these cranial nerves have both sensory and motor neurons, although some of them have only motor neurons.

The twelve different cranial nerves are:

- The adduced nerve
- The accessory nerve
- The facial nerve
- The glossopharyngeal nerve
- The hypoglossal nerve
- The oculomotor nerve
- The olfactory nerve
- The optic nerve
- The trigeminal nerve
- The trochlear nerve
- The vagus nerve
- The vestibular-nuclear nerve

The olfactory nerve CN1

The first cranial nerve is called the olfactory nerve. The first cranial nerve contains sensory nerves related to the sense of smell. The olfactory nerve has major olfactory receptor neurons located in the upper part of the nasal cavity. The olfactory nerve is made up of grouped nerve fibers and these fibers are excited by molecules in the air. The fibers sends this signal to the olfactory bulb which then transmits the information to the brain.

The optic nerve

The optic nerve is a coupled nerve, one for each side of the body, which is responsible for transmitting information about visual stimuli to the brain. The visual information that is collected from the various parts of the eye, such as rods and cones, is transported through the optic nerve through the occipital lobe of the brain. The optic nerve is also liable for facilitating the focusing of the eye on objects and narrowing the pupil in response to light.

The oculomotor nerve

The third cranial nerve, the oculomotor nerve, is important for managing most of the eye's movement. It also allows the eyelids to rise. The oculomotor nerve has general somatic efferent axons (GSE) that are responsible for managing the movement of various skeletal muscle groups around the eye such as the upper recti and upper eyelids.

The trochlear nerve

The fourth one in the cranial nerve is the trochlear nerve. The troclear nerve has only somatic motor components. The service of the trochlear nerve is to innervate the superior oblique muscle, which is located in the region surrounding the eye. It allows precise eye movements when tracking objects.

The trigeminal nerve

The trigeminal nerve is split into three different branches, making it the largest nerve of all the cranial nerves. The trigeminal nerve is the major sensory nerve of the face. Not only does it provide sensory information on the face, but it also plays a vital role in enabling functions such as chewing and biting.

The abducens nerve

Many nerves are involved in the functioning of the eyeball due to how complex it is. The abducens nerve, the sixth cranial nerve, helps to move the rectus muscle of the laterus of the eye. This means that it is involved in directing the eye's gaze outward or away from the nostril.

The facial nerve

The seventh cranial nerve is the facial nerve. The facial nerve, as the name suggests, deals with facial movement. The facial nerve allows the wide variety of facial expressions that man has innervating all the various muscles of the face, such as the procero muscle and nose. The facial nerve also carries a great deal of sensory information to the brain, including information relating to taste.

The vestibular-nuclear nerve

The eighth cranial nerve, AKA, the vestibular-nuclear nerve, is responsible for transmitting information about sound to the brain. The sensory cells of the ear detect information, which is then transported along the vestibular-nuclear nerve. The vestibular-cochlear nerve is a combination of the vestibular nerve that carries information on balance and the cochlear nerve that carries auditory information.

The glossopharyngeal nerve

Here the upper parts of the glossopharyngeal nerve, vagus nerve and accessory nerve are visible.

The glossopharyngeal nerve is the ninth cranial nerve and has a number of different functions concerning the nose, mouth, and throat. The glossopharyngeal nerve takes information from the middle ear, the tonsils, and the back of the tongue. It also receives sensory messages from the carotid bodies and allows the pharyngeal plexus to move.

The vagus nerve

The vagus nerve is the tenth one in the cranial nerve. The vagus nerve descends from the skull to the core of the body where it interfaces with the digestive tract, the heart and the lungs through a series of different sections. The different sections make the vagus nerve the cranial nerve with the greatest distribution. The vagus nerve supplies the parasympathetic motor fibers to almost all the organs of the body. The vagus nerve controls a series of skeletal muscles including the palatoglossus muscle and the cricothyroid muscle.

The accessory nerve

The accessory nerve, sometimes called the accessory spinal cranial nerve, controls two muscles in the upper part of the body. The accessory nerve is involved in the movement of the sternocleidomastoid muscle, which allows the head to turn. The accessory nerve is also important for the movement of the trapezius muscle, which allows it to move and shrug the shoulders. The portion of the accessory nerve inside the skull provides motor control to the muscles of the pharynx and larynx.

The hypoglossal nerve

The hypoglossal nerve is the twelfth and final cranial nerve, and it is responsible for the innervation of the internal and external tongue muscles. The nerve helps the muscles to move and slide out from the tongue, although this nerve has only a motor function. The nerve allows you to do the wide range of tongue movements needed to eat, drink, speak and clean your mouth.

Damage to any of these nerves can cause a number of problems, such as facial paralysis or difficulty in speaking.

The cranial nerves, allows us to be able to do the various movements necessary to stay alive.

Summary of the 12 Cranial Nerves

CN I	Olfactory nerve	Smell	helps to locate food
CN II	Optic nerve	Vision	makes it possible to see
CN III	Oculomotor nerve	Looking	controls some eyeball muscles
CN IV	Trochlear nerve	Looking	controls some eyeball muscles
CN V	Trigeminal nerve	Chewing and swallowing Hearing	tensor tympani muscle
CN VI	Abducens nerve	Looking	controls some eyeball muscles
CN VII	Facial nerve secretions	Chewing	some facial muscles and saliva Hearing; stapedius muscle
CN VIII	Acoustic nerve	Hearing	translates sound waves into nerve
CN IX	Glossopharyngeal nerve	Swallowing	
CN X	The new (ventral) vagus branch		innervates and controls the upper third of the esophagus and most of the pharyngeal muscles, it regulates the heart and bronchi.
	Old vagus nerve	The old (dorsal) vagus branch	innervates the lower two thirds of the esophagus; it regulates the stomach function, digestive glands and organs such as liver and gall bladder, and movement

			of food through the intestines (except the descending colon).
CN XI	Spinal accessory nerve		Innervates the trapezius and sternocleidomastoid muscles which turn the head and expand the visual field
CN XII	Hypoglossal nerve		Moves the tongue

In addition to eating, cranial nerves perform other functions. The visceral afferent (sensory) branches of the cranial nerves V, VII, IX, X, and XI collect information from our visceral organs: are we safe, threatened, or in danger of death? Does our body feel healthy, or is there an imbalance, pain, dysfunction, or illness? If we are safe and sound, these nerves facilitate the desirable state of social commitment.

CHAPTER 3

CRANIAL NERVE DYSFUNCTION AND SOCIAL COMMITMENT

We believe that "normal" human behavior is an expression of positive social values. Our actions must be useful for our survival and well-being, as well as for the well-being of others.

When we are socially engaged, it is easy for other people to understand our behavior and what we do makes sense to others; most of us are socially engaged most of the time. However, sometimes we temporarily fall into a state of chronic activation of the spinal sympathetic chain system (fighting or flight) or vagal dorsal activity (withdrawal, arrest). So, if our autonomic nervous system is resistant, we will soon return to a state of social commitment.

Unfortunately, most of us are not socially active most of the time. If we lack the necessary resistance to return spontaneously to a state of social commitment, we are trapped in the sympathetic chain or in the vagal dorsal states. In these states, it is often difficult for other people to understand our values, motivation and behavior. Our actions seem irrational, often go against our interests and can be destructive for us and others. If we do not commit ourselves socially, life becomes difficult, not only for ourselves but also for those around us.

Let's take a look at the five cranial nerves needed for social participation and what kind of problems can arise when they don't work properly. These symptoms provide an indication that someone is not socially engaged; a person with these symptoms can benefit from the treatment of the affected nerves.

FIFTH AND SEVENTH CRANIAN NERVES

CN V, the trigeminal nerve, has various motor functions, including the control of the masticatory muscles that move the jaw when we chew. CN V also has sensory functions and receives impulses from the sensory nerves of the facial skin.

CN VII, the facial nerve, also possess several motor functions. Check the tension and relaxation of the individual muscles of the face. Changes in the pattern of tension in the facial muscles create our facial expressions, which not only communicate different emotions but also reflect our internal states in terms of health or illness. Ideally, changes in facial expressions are spontaneous and reflect the flow of changes in emotions and thoughts.

Is someone's face expressionless, lacking in animation? This is usually a sign of CN VII dysfunction. We can make a voluntary grimace, for example, smile or open our eyes. But these are not the same as spontaneous facial expressions.

Small spontaneous changes in the facial expression (or lack thereof) in this transverse strip from the corners of the eyes to the corners of the lips, if others notice consciously or unconsciously, can reveal whether we are socially engaged or not.

In addition to these separate functions, CN V and CN VII have related functions. CN VII innervates the muscles of the face and CN V is a sensory nerve of the facial skin. When we change the facial expression, this gives us the "feeling of the face". Both nerves play a role in listening and understanding what is being said, allowing us to participate in a conversation. This is also essential to facilitate social engagement.

Stapedium, the smallest muscle in the body, is innervated by the CN VII. This muscle protects the inner ear from high noise levels, mainly the volume of one's voice. The roar of a lion can be deafening, causing terror to other animals to the point of paralyzing them. The lion protects itself from the sound of its own voice by crushing its stapedium muscle a moment before roaring, so that it is not affected by the loud noise.

By reducing the volume of sounds above and below the frequency of the human female voice, the stapedium muscle allows the child to hear his mother's voice more clearly. If the background noise disturbs you easily, the stapedius muscle may not do its job in reducing the volume of low-frequency sounds, making it difficult to hear what someone else is saying in a noisy room.

Hyperacusis, another hearing problem, may be the result of dysfunction of the stapedium and other muscles of the middle ear, the tympanic tensor or the tympanic muscle innervated by CN V. As these muscles become stiff, the tension increases, decreasing the sound. This is a useful function when we eat, reducing the level of chewing noise.

CN V and CN VII dysfunctions are quite common in adults, often as an undesirable side effect of dental extractions or orthodontic appliances. I have taken note in many of my clients who have had dental work that the pterygoid process of their sphenoid and palatine bone (one of the small facial bones) on their hard palate is "extracted from the joint" in relation to each other. As part of my training in craniosacral biomechanical therapy, I learned to observe the shape of the hard palate to see if the palatine bone moved sideways and to perform a technique to bring this bone back to its lateral side and perform a technique to return this bone in the correct position.

Some of the branches of CN V and CN VII are located in this area. A very slight misalignment of the facial bones in the joint between the sphenoids and the palatine bones can put pressure on both nerves. Sometimes I treat patients who have had problems with these two nerves after extracting a tooth. When I ask the dentists about the pain of a tooth and the misalignment of these two bones, most of them know exactly what I mean. They often respond by being very careful not to remove a tooth just because of pain if there are no signs of infection.

The sphenoid bone is the most central bone in the skull. The outer surfaces of the sphenoid bone form what we commonly call the temples. If a boxer is hit in one of the temples, he risks being eliminated. Many boxers know this and attack their opponent's temples. If they hit the temple, they will definitely win by knockout. This is also the reason why baseball hitters wear a cap with lapels that protect their temples from injury if hit by a ball. The innermost part of the sphenoid bone has a saddle-shaped depression in which the pituitary gland rests.

When a branch of a cranial nerve is under direct physical pressure, not only that branch but other branches of that nerve can become dysfunctional. Therefore, a dislocation between the sphenoids and the palatine bones can cause dysfunction of the nerves of the face and middle ear. This is sufficient to block the entire nervous system of social commitment.

The cranial nerve V goes to the skin of the face, while the cranial nerve VII goes to the muscles of the face. To correct some of these dysfunctions and give oneself a natural "facelift," the second part of this book includes a technique that stimulates the fifth and seventh cranial nerves. Although you should notice an improvement in the reduction of facial tensions the first time you train, it is a good idea to repeat it occasionally, especially if you have lost your natural smile because you are in a sympathetic vagal or spinal dorsal state.

Two other muscles innervated by CN V are the medial and lateral pterygoids, which occur in the sphenoid bone and help to open and close the jaw. A slight shift of this bone can cause irregularities such as excessive bite, under bite or cross bite.

THE NINTH, TENTH AND ELEVENTH CRANIAL NERVES

One of the two sections of the tenth cranial nerve (the ventral vagus) rises in a structure called the ambiguous nucleus in the brain stem, together with the ninth and the eleventh cranial nerves.

The dorsal part of the vagus nerve originates on the floor of the fourth ventricle near the posterior part in the brainstem. (The ventricle is not a physical structure, but it is a space between the lobes of the brain, filled with cerebrospinal fluid. There are four of these ventricles, connected together through small channels.)

The two branches of the vagus nerve, along with the ninth and the eleventh cranial nerves and the jugular vein, pass through the jugular hole, a small opening at the base of the skull between the temporal and occipital bones.

The ninth and eleventh cranial nerve fibers intertwine with the tenth cranial nerve fiber. My anatomy professor, Professor Pat Coughlin, told our class that in modern interpretations of anatomy, a growing number of professors consider CN IX and CN X as two parts of the same nerve. Just as nerve fibers intertwine, their functionality appears to be related as components of the nervous system of social engagement.

For the clinical purposes of bringing the nervous system into a state of social commitment, I find it easier to turn to the ninth, tenth and eleventh cranial nerves as if they were a single nerve. When a patient has symptoms that indicate dysfunction in one, there is almost always dysfunction in the other two. If, after treatment, the patient shows an improvement in the vagal function test (CN X), generally the symptoms attributed to the ninth and eleventh cranial nerve dysfunction also disappear.

NINTH CRANIAL NERVE

The ninth cranial nerve is called the glossopharyngeal nerve (glosso - refers to the tongue and pharyngeal to the pharynx, the back of the upper part of the throat). This nerve has efferent (motor) and afferent (sensory) fibers. The efferent part innervates a single muscle, the styloopharynx-geo, which assists to swallow.

The ninth cranial nerve collects sensory information from the tonsils, the pharynx, the middle ear and the posterior third of the tongue. It is also a part of the mechanism of regulation of blood pressure: it has afferent branches in the carotid sinus, located at the base of the neck near the carotid arteries, and its sensory fibers control blood pressure to influence the heart and blood, toning the muscle cells in the arteries.

This nerve also controls the levels of oxygen and carbon dioxide in the blood to regulate the respiratory rate. It is also responsible for stimulating the secretion of the parotid gland, the large salivary gland in front of the ear.

THE TENTH CRANIAL NERVE (THE VAGUS)

The tenth cranial nerve plays a vital part in the autonomic nervous system. Before Stephen Porges presented the polyvagal theory, the poodle had to function as a single neural pathway. However, we now know that the two branches of the vagus, ventral and dorsal nerve arise in different places and have very different functions, and this book has been written to clarify those differences and their implications.

THE BRANCH OF SUBDIAPHRAGMATIC VAGUS (DORSAL)

The dorsal branch of the vagus nerve posseses motor fibers that innervate the visceral organs below the respiratory diaphragm: stomach, liver, spleen, kidneys, gall bladder, urinary bladder, small intestine, pancreas, and ascending and transverse compartment of the colon. Therefore, this branch has sometimes been refer to as the "subdiaphragmatic branch of the vagus nerve".

However, this description is only partially accurate, since some fibers that originate in the dorsal motor nucleus of the brain stem also influence the heart and the lungs, which are located above the diaphragm. Likewise, although the ventral vagus primarily supplies motor pathways to the organs above the diaphragm, some fibers affect the organs below the diaphragm. The three parts of the autonomic nervous system, the dorsal and ventral branches of the vagus nerve, and the spinal system, the dorsal and ventral branches of the vagus nerve and the sympathetic spinal chain, influence the vital functions of respiration and blood circulation. Each of the three circuits affects the heart and lungs in different ways.

The appendix includes two drawings of the visceral organs. One shows those innervated by the ventral vagus and the other shows those innervated by the dorsal vagus.

OTHER FUNCTIONS OF THE VENTRAL BRANCH OF THE VAGUS NERVE

The ventral branch of the vagus nerve emanates from the brain stem, in the upper part of the spinal cord under the brain. It stimulates the rhythmic constriction of the bronchioles, facilitating the extraction of oxygen, while the area of the brainstem that controls the vagal dorsal activation can cause a chronic constriction of the airways, which makes the passage of air difficult. (This is part of the mechanism that activates in a state of arrest or shock. The narrowing of the bronchioles also occurs in COPD, chronic bronchitis and asthma.)

When we feel safe, the ventral branch of the vagus nerve favors rest or quiet activity. There is a rhythmic hesitation of the airway opening; they are moderately open by inhalation and moderately closed by inhalation.

The ventral branch of the vagus nerve innervates a lot of the small muscles of the throat, including the vocal cords, the larynx, the pharynx and some muscles in the back of the pharynx.

THE ELEVENTH CRANIAL NERVE

The eleventh cranial nerve, referred to as the "accessory nerve", is one of the keys to the well-being of the entire musculoskeletal system. Since it traps the trapezius and sternocleidomastoid (SCM) muscles, which allow movement of the head and neck, the tension in one of these muscles on one side pushes the shoulder, the spine and the entire body out of alignment.

Both the trapezius and the sternocleidomastoid muscles originate in the bones of the skull. (The trapezius adheres to the mastoid process of the temporal bone and of the sternocleidomastoid to the occipital bone.) Together they form the outer ring of the neck, shoulder and upper back muscles.

If the eleventh cranial nerve is dysfunctional, it results in a lack of adequate tone in these muscles. This in turn can cause acute or chronic shoulder problems, stiff neck, headache and difficulty turning the head to one side. (See chapter 5 for more information on these muscles. The second part also contains a treatment to relieve migraine by reducing excessive tension in these muscles.)

Instead of simply massaging a trapezoidal or chronically flaccid or flaccid SCM muscle, it is best for a therapist to first improve the function of the eleventh cranial nerve using the basic exercise and then massage the muscles after the nerve works again.

SPINAL NERVES

Most people have heard of problems resulting from spinal nerve dysfunction. Many people suffer from a herniated disc that presses the spinal cord or a bone growth (spinal stenosis) that can press on a spinal nerve and cause pain, loss of sensation or loss of function (for example, bladder control). Spinal nerve dysfunction can also cause local paralysis (inability to use a specific skeletal muscle).

Some people use chiropractic or osteopathic treatments to relieve spinal cord compression. Chiropractors generally use high-speed and short-push techniques to reposition a vertebra, aligning it better and removing pressure from the pain-causing nerve. Osteopaths have the same goal, but generally use a softer approach.

Other popular "conservative" treatments for the spine include yoga and stretching, strengthening the back muscles with calisthenics, weight training, physiotherapy and massages to balance the tone of the back muscles. If these methods fail to keep the spine in shape, we may feel invalidated, dejected, and inclined to choose radical treatments such as surgery.

Back surgery is a booming business. About 500,000 Americans undergo surgery every year just for problems with their lower back. Unfortunately, surgery does not always buy relief. And studies show that most back pains go away on their own in time.

For decades, orthopedic surgeons have treated back problems by cutting off part of a protruding disc, cutting a bone spur or even inserting a metal plate and screws to harden the adjacent vertebrae. Despite the widespread use of surgery, the effectiveness of these operations is not scientifically documented. On the contrary, there is more and more research showing that these operations are not effective in the long term.

An important function of the spinal nerves is to allow us to use our arms, legs and trunk to move our body by contracting and relaxing different muscles. The spinal nerves also innervate some visceral organs. Spinal nerve messages come from the brain and travel through the spinal cord, a bundle of nerves in the form of a tube that leaves the skull through a large opening at the base of the skull called the foramen magnum (in Latin, "big hole").

After leaving the skull, the pairs of spinal nerves emanate from the spinal cord, emerging through the spaces between the adjacent vertebrae to serve the muscles, joints, ligaments, tendons, internal organs and skin. Humans have thirty-three pairs of spinal nerves, with one nerve for each pair that goes to the right side of the body and the other to the left.

Each pair of spinal nerves corresponds to a segment of the spine. There are thirty-three vertebrae in total: seven in the neck, twelve in the thorax, five in the lumbar region, five in the sacrum and four in the coccyx. The spinal nerves, which include the motor and sensory nerves, carry round-trip signals between the brain and the rest of the body. Two important exceptions are the trapezius and sternocleidomastoid muscles in the neck and shoulder, which receive their innervation from the eleventh cranial nerve.

There is always more than one branch of a spinal nerve that goes to a given muscle. This provides the assurance that if one of the spinal nerves is damaged, the muscle can still work (albeit less efficiently) using signals from other available nerves.

Each spinal nerve also affects different muscles. Often the muscles are part of a chain of movement. For example, the muscles of the shoulder, upper arm, forearm, wrist and fingers work together as a unit to control the basic movements of the arm or hand.

The motor pathways of a nerve tell a muscle to contract. The spinal sensory nerves collect various types of information from the body and return it to the brain: they bring feelings of pain, positions of the parts of the body in relation to each other, movement, tension in the muscles or in the band and sense of touch for the whole body, except the face (which is innervated by the cranial nerves).

The branches of the spinal and cranial nerves are traditionally classified in sensory and motor functions; truely this is oversimplification. If we asses the individual "motor nerves" more closely, we observe that some of their fibers are motor fibers, but that they also contain sensory fibers that report the state of tension of a muscle to the brain. We now know that most of the fibers in the "motor nerves" are sensory also.

This combination of motor and sensory nerve fibers provides a feedback circuit that allows us to use the motor fibers to tighten a muscle, while the sensory fibers simultaneously send information to the brain about the change in tension level in the muscle. This allows us to calibrate the muscle tension, a much more powerful and efficient approach than the fact that the muscle can be completely stretched or not, which would be the case if we did not have feedback from the sensory fiber.

In normal conditions, the spinal nerves facilitate easy, well-coordinated and elegant movements, and the muscles are activated using minimum amount of energy to accomplish the desired motion. However, if the body is in a position of stress and all the muscles are more tense than necessary, this natural coordination is often lost and the movements become uncoordinated, uncomfortable or weak.

THE SPINAL SYMPATHIC CHAIN

The spinal nerve branches go to specific body structures: skin (dermatomes), muscles (myotomes), visceral organs (viscerotomes) and ligaments, fascia and connective tissue (fasciatomas). Instead of a single spinal nerve that innervates a single muscle, there is some overlap, so that the branches of different spinal nerves can innervate the same single muscle. This creates a backup system so that if one part of a nerve is damaged, other parts can still contract the same muscle and can still work, even if it works less efficiently.

A few of the spinal nerves go to the internal organs. For example, the nerves of the thoracic vertebrae T1 and T4 go to the heart, the nerves of T5 and T8 go to the lungs, T9 goes to the stomach and T10 goes to the kidneys. Other nerves serve other structures, such as the bladder, genitals and intestines.

Upon exiting the spinal cord, some thoracic and upper lumbar spinal nerve fibers (T1 - L2) extend laterally a short distance. While some remain in the same area, others join the fibers of the vertebrae up and down to be part of the sympathetic chain. The sympathetic chain extends along the spine between T1 and L2, connecting to these spinal nerves. Most of the sympathetic, which project towards the visceral organs and the head, are accompanied by arteries towards their destination.

When we face a risk to our survival, there is an increase in the activity of the whole sympathetic chain, extending the fight or flight response to mobilize the whole body's resources. This response is instant and total, which is appropriate if we are threatened or in danger. Tense muscles to prepare for the movements needed to fight or flee; This is described in weight lifting circles as "pumping".

The organs innervated by these sympathetic nerve fibers increase their activity level to support this movement. For example, the heart beats quicker to supply more blood to the muscular system. Blood pressure increases to be able to release more blood to tense muscles. The liver releases sugars stored in the blood so that extra energy is available to burn the muscles. The response to the survival stress of the sympathetic chain causes the airway muscles to open to the fullest, improving our respiratory capacity and absorbing the maximum amount of oxygen to mobilize completely to fight or run.

At the same time, other organs (mainly those involved in digestion) slow down or stop. There is a decrease in appetite, the movement of food in the intestine slows down or stops and the person may experience a "butterfly" sensation in the stomach.

In the event of a threat or challenge, the state of stress created by the sympathetic response affects the whole body and can simultaneously involve the muscles of all segments. Activation of the spinal sympathetic chain in the "fight or flight" response is one of the three possible states of the autonomic nervous system, which will be discussed in more detail below.

THE ENTERIC NERVOUS SYSTEM

The enteric nervous system is also a network of nerves that interconnect the visceral organs. We know almost nothing about these nerves; Since they are so intertwined with each other, with the visceral organs and with the connective tissue between the organs, it has so far been impossible for the anatomists to completely trace the enteric nerve pathways.

Furthermore, we know almost nothing about how enteric nerves work. At best, we can assume that the enteric nerves somehow help the various visceral organs to communicate with each other to coordinate the complex process of digestion.

The enteric nervous system is sometimes also called "the second brain", which has an intelligence that works beyond our consciousness. We cannot consciously know what is going on in our digestive process or regulate it voluntarily.

CHAPTER 4

THE VAGUS NERVE

The vagus nerve is the primary component of the parasympathetic nervous system, which oversees a wide range of crucial bodily functions, including mood control, immune response, heart rate and digestion. It establishes one of the networks between the brain and the gastrointestinal tract and sends information on the state of internal organs to the brain through afferent fibers. In this chapter, we discuss various functions of the vagus nerve that make it an attractive target in the treatment of psychiatric and gastrointestinal disorders. Preliminary evidence exists that vagus nerve stimulation is a promising additional treatment for treatment-refractory depression, post-traumatic stress disorder and inflammatory bowel disease. Treatments that affect the vagus nerve increase vagal tone and inhibit the production of cytokines. Both are important resilience mechanisms. Stimulation of the vagal afferent fibers in the intestine influences the monoaminergic brain systems in the brainstem that play crucial roles in the main psychiatric conditions, such as mood and anxiety disorders. Online, there is preliminary evidence for intestinal bacteria to have beneficial effects on mood and anxiety, in part by influencing vagus nerve activity.

Because vagal tone is related to the ability to regulate stress responses and may be affected by breathing, its increase through meditation and yoga probably contributes to resilience and mitigation of mood and anxiety symptoms.

BASIC ANATOMY OF THE VAGUS NERVE

The vagus nerve carries a wide range of signals from the digestive system and organs to the brain and vice versa. It is the tenth cranial nerve, which extends from its origin in the brainstem through the neck and chest to the abdomen. Because of its long journey through the human body, it has also been described as the "wandering nerve".

The vagus nerve leaves the medulla oblongata in the groove between the olives and the inferior cerebellar peduncle, leaving the skull through the central compartment of the jugular foramen. In the neck, the vagus nerve provides innervation necessary to most of the pharynx and larynx muscles, which are responsible for swallowing and vocalization. In the chest, it provides the main parasympathetic contribution to the heart and stimulates a reduction in heart rate. In the intestine, the vagus nerve regulates the contraction of smooth muscles and glandular secretion. The preganglionic neurons of the vagal efferent fibers emerge from the dorsal motor nucleus of the vagus nerve located in the medulla, and innervate the muscular and mucous layers of the intestine, both in the lamina propria and in the external musculature. The celiac branch supplies the intestine from the duodenum proximal to the distal part of the descending colon. Abdominal vagal afferents include chemoreceptors, mucosal mechanoreceptors, and tension receptors in the esophagus, the stomach and the proximal small intestine and sensory terminations in the liver and pancreas. Sensory afferent cellular bodies are found in the nodose ganglia and send information to the solitary tractus nucleus (NTS). NTS projects vagal sensory information in different regions of the central nervous system, such as the locus coeruleus (LC), the ventrolateral rostral marrow, the amygdala and the thalamus.

The vagus nerve is responsible for regulating the internal functions of organs, such as digestion, heart rate and respiratory rate, as well as vasomotor activity and some reflex actions, such as coughing, sneezing, swallowing and vomiting. Its invigoration leads to the release of acetylcholine (ACh) in the synaptic junction with secreting cells, intrinsic nerve fibers and smooth muscles. ACh fasten to nicotinic and muscarinic receptors and stimulates muscle contractions in the parasympathetic nervous system.

Animal studies have shown a remarkable capacity for regeneration of the vagus nerve. For example, subdiaframatic vagotomy induced transient withdrawal and restoration of central vagal afferents, as well as synaptic plasticity in NTS. Furthermore, regeneration of vagal afferents in rats can be achieved 18 weeks after subdiaphragmatic vagotomy, although efferent re-innervation of the gastrointestinal tract is not restored even after 45 weeks.

THE ROLE OF VAGUS IN THE FUNCTIONS OF THE AUTONOMIC NERVOUS SYSTEM

Besides the enteric nervous system (ENS) and the sympathetic nervous system, the parasympathetic nervous system serves one of the three sections of the autonomic nervous system.

The definition of the parasympathetic and sympathetic nervous system is mainly anatomical. The vagus nerve is the primary contributor of the parasympathetic nervous system. Three other parasympathetic cranial nerves are the oculomotor nerve, the facial nerve and the glossopharyngeal nerve.

The most essential function of the vagus nerve is afferent, bringing information to the internal organs, such as intestines, liver, heart and lungs to the brain. This suggests that internal organs are the main sources of sensory information for the brain. The intestine is the largest surface towards the outside world and could therefore be a particularly vital sensory organ.

Historically, the vagus has been examined as an efferent nerve and as an opposite of the sympathetic nervous system. Most organs receive parasympathetic efferents from the vagus nerve and sympathetic efferents through the splanchnic nerves. Together with the sympathetic nervous system, the parasympathetic nervous system is responsible for regulating vegetative functions by acting in mutual opposition. Parasympathetic innervation causes dilation of blood vessels and bronchioles and stimulation of the salivary glands. On the other side, the sympathetic innervation leads to a tightening of the blood vessels, a dilation of the bronchioles, an increase in heart rate and a constriction of the intestinal and urinary sphincters. In the gastrointestinal tract, activation of the parasympathetic nervous system increases intestinal motility and glandular secretion. On the contrary, sympathetic activity leads to a reduction in intestinal activity and a reduction in blood flow to the intestine, allowing a higher blood flow to the heart and muscles, when the individual faces existential stress.

The ENS derives from neural crest cells of mainly vagal origin and consists of a nerve plexus embedded in the intestinal wall, which extends over the entire gastrointestinal tract from the esophagus to the anus. It is estimated that human ENS have about 100-500 million neurons. This is the largest concentration of nerve cells in the human body. Since ENS is similar to the brain in terms of structure, function and chemical coding, it has been described as "the second brain" or "the brain in the intestine". It consists of two ganglionic plexuses: the submucosal plexus, which regulates the gastrointestinal blood flow and controls the functions and the secretion of epithelial cells and the myenteric plexus, which mainly regulates relaxation and contraction of the intestinal wall. ENS acts as an intestinal barrier and regulates the main enteric processes, such as the immune response, nutrient detection, motility, microvascular circulation and epithelial secretion of fluids, ions and bioactive peptides.

There is clearly a "communication" between the vagal nerve and the ENS and the main transmitter is cholinergic activation through nicotinic receptors. The interaction of ENS and the vagal nerve as part of the central nervous system leads to a two-way transmission of instruction. So also, the ENS in the large intestine is also able to function quite independently of vagal control as it contains complete reflex circuits, including sensory neurons and motor neurons. They regulate muscle activity and motility, fluid flows, mucosal blood flow and also the mucosal barrier function. ENS neurons are also in close contact with the cells of the adaptive and innate immune system and regulate their functions and activities. Aging and cell loss in ENS are associated with disorders such as constipation, incontinence and evacuation disorders. The loss of ENS in the small and large intestine can be life-threatening (Hirschsprung's disease; intestinal pseudo-obstruction).

VAGUS NERVE AS A LINK BETWEEN THE CNS AND ENS

Relations between CNS and ENS, also known as the brain-intestine axis, allows the bidirectional connection between the brain and the gastrointestinal tract. It is responsible for monitoring physiological homeostasis and connecting the emotional and cognitive areas of the brain with peripheral intestinal functions, such as immune activation, intestinal permeability, enteric reflex and enteroendocrine signaling. This brain-gut axis includes the brain, spinal cord, autonomic nervous system (sympathetic, parasympathetic and ENS) and the hypothalamic-pituitary-adrenal axis (HPA). The vagal efferents directs the signals "down" from the brain to the intestine through the efferent fibers, which represent 10-20% of all the fibers and the vagal afferents "up" from the intestinal wall to the brain which represent 80-90% of all the fibers. The vagal afferent paths are involved in the activation/regulation of the HPA axis, which coordinates the body's adaptive responses to stress factors of any kind. Environmental stress and elevated systemic proinflammatory cytokines activate the HPA axis through the secretion of corticotropin release factor (CRF) from the hypothalamus. The release of CRF stimulates the secretion of the adrenocorticotropic hormone (ACTH) from the pituitary gland. This stimulation, in turn, leads to the release of cortisol from the adrenal glands. Cortisol is an important stress hormone that affects many human organs, including the brain, bones, muscles and body fat.

Both neural (vague) and hormonal (HPA axis) lines of communication combine to allow the brain to influence the activities of intestinal functional effector cells, such as immune cells, epithelial cells, enteric neurons, smooth muscle cells, interstitial cells of Cajal and enterochromaffin cells. These cells, are under the influence of intestinal microbiota. Intestinal microbiota has an important impact on the brain-intestine axis, interacting not only locally with intestinal cells and ENS, but also directly influencing neuroendocrine and metabolic systems. Emerging data support the role of the microbiota in influencing anxiety and depressive behaviors (34). Studies conducted on germ-free animals have shown that microbiota influences stress reactivity and anxiety-like behavior and regulates the HPA activity set point. Therefore, these animals generally show reduced anxiety (35) and increased stress response with increased levels of ACTH and cortisol.

In the case of food intake, the vagal afferents that innervate the gastrointestinal tract provide a quick and discreet account of digestible food and circulating and stored fuels, while the vagal efferents along with hormonal mechanisms encode the rate of absorption, storage and mobilization of nutrients. Histological and electrophysiological evidence reveals that visceral afferent nerve endings in the intestinal nerve express a wide range of chemical and mechanosensitive receptors. These receptors are targets of intestinal hormones and regulatory peptides that are released by enteroendocrine cells of the gastrointestinal system in response to nutrients, stomach distension and neuronal signals. They direct the control of food intake and the regulation of satiety, gastric emptying and energy balance by transmitting the signals that arise from the upper intestine to the core of the solitary tract in the brain. Most of these hormones, such as cholecystokinin peptide (CCK), ghrelin and leptin are sensitive to the nutrient content in the intestine and are involved in the regulation of short-term feelings of hunger and satiety.

Cholecystokinin regulates the gastrointestinal functions, including inhibition of gastric emptying and food intake through the activation of CCK-1 receptors on the vagal afferent fibers that innervate the intestine. Furthermore, CCK is important for the secretion of pancreatic fluid and the production of gastric acid, the contraction of the gallbladder, the reduction of gastric emptying and digestion. Saturated fats, long chain fatty acids, amino acids and small peptides that result from protein digestion stimulate the release of CCK from the small intestine.

There are different biologically active forms of CCK, classified according to the number of amino acids they contain, for example CCK-5, CCK-8, CCK-22 and CCK-33. In neurons, CCK-8 is always the predominant form, while endocrine intestinal cells contain a mixture of small and larger CCK peptides of which CCK-33 or CCK-22 often prevail. In rats, both long-chain fatty acids and short-chain fatty acids activate fasting vagal afferent nerve fibers, but do so with distinct mechanisms. Short chain fatty acids, such as butyric acid, have a direct effect on the vagal afferent end groups while long chain fatty acids activate vagal afferents through a CCK-dependent mechanism.

Exogenous CCK administration appears to inhibit the endogenous CCK secretion. CCK can aslo be found in enteric vagal afferent neurons, in the cerebral cortex, in the thalamus, in the hypothalamus, in the basal ganglia and in dorsal weakening and functions as a neurotransmitter. It directly activates the vagal afferent terminals in the NTS increasing the release of calcium. Furthermore, there is evidence that CCK can activate neurons in the navel and in the intestinal myenteric plexus (a plexus that provides motor innervation to both layers of the muscular layer of the intestine), in rats and that treatment with vagotomy or capsaicin causes an attenuation of the CCK expression of Fos induced (a type of proto-oncogene) in the brain. There is also substantial evidence that elevated CCK levels induce feelings of anxiety. Therefore, CCK is used as a challenging agent to model anxiety disorders in humans and animals.

Ghrelin is another hormone released into circulation by the stomach and plays a key role in stimulating food intake by inhibiting the vagal afferent fire. Circulating ghrelin levels increase fasting and decrease after a meal. Central or peripheral administration of ghrelin acylated in rats strongly stimulates food intake and the release of growth hormone and chronic administration causes weight gain. The action of ghrelin on nutrition is abolished or attenuated in rats subjected to vagotomy or treatment with capsaicin, a specific afferent neurotoxin. With humans, intravenous infusion or subcutaneous injection increases the sensation of hunger and food intake, as ghrelin suppresses the release of insulin. Therefore, it is not surprising that the secretion is disturbed in obesity and insulin resistance.

Leptin receptors have also been ascertained in the vagus nerve. Rodent studies clearly indicate that leptin and CCK interact synergistically to induce short-term inhibition of food intake and long-term reduction in body weight. The epithelial cells that react to both ghrelin and leptin are located near the vagal mucosal ends and modulate the activity of the vagal afferents, acting in concert to regulate food intake. After fasting and diet-induced obesity in mice, leptin loses its potentiating effect on the afferents of the vagal mucosa.

The gastrointestinal pathway is the major interface between food and the human body and can perceive basic tastes in much the same way as the tongue, through the use of taste receptors similar to associated G proteins. Different taste qualities induce the release of different gastric peptides. Bitter taste receptors can be considered as potential targets for reducing hunger by stimulating the release of CCK. Furthermore, the activation of the bitter taste receptors stimulates the secretion of ghrelin and, therefore, influences the vagus nerve.

VAGUS NERVE AS MODULATOR OF INTESTINAL IMMUNE HOMEOSTASIS

The gastrointestinal tract is constantly bombarded with food antigens, possible pathogens and symbiotic intestinal microbiota that present a risk factor for intestinal inflammation. It is strongly innervated by the vagal fibers that connect the central nervous system to the intestinal immune system, making the vagus an important component, the neuroendocrine-immune axis. This axis is involved in coordinated neuronal, behavioral and endocrine responses that are important for first-line defense against inflammation. For example, in response to pathogens and other harmful stimuli, the tumor alpha-necrosis factor (TNF-α), a cytokine, is produced by activated macrophages, dendritic cells and other mucosal cells. Together with prostaglandins and interferons, TNF-α is an important mediator of local and systemic inflammation and increases cause the cardinal clinical signs of inflammation, including heat, swelling, pain and redness. Counter-regulatory mechanisms such as immunologically competent cells and anti-inflammatory cytokines normally limit the acute inflammatory response and prevent the spread of inflammatory mediators in the blood stream. Furthermore, there is a "wired" connection between the functions of the nervous system and the immune system as an anti-inflammatory mechanism. The vagal dorsal complex, including the sensory nuclei of the solitary tract, the postrema area and the dorsal motor nucleus of the vagus, responds to the increase in circulating amounts of TNF-α by altering the motor activity in the vagus nerve.

The anti-inflammatory abilities of the vagus nerve are mediated through three different routes. The first path is the HPA axis, which was described above. The second way is the splenic sympathetic anti-inflammatory pathway, in which the vagus nerve stimulates the splenic sympathetic nerve. The norepinephrine (NE) (noradrenaline) released at the distal end of the splenic nerve connects to the $\beta2$ adrenergic receptor of the splenic lymphocytes that release ACh. Finally, ACh inhibits TNF-α release by spleen macrophages via α-7-nicotinic ACh receptors. The last route, called the cholinergic anti-inflammatory route (CAIP), is mediated by vagal efferent fibers that synapse on enteric neurons, which in turn release ACh to the synaptic junction with macrophages. ACh binds to the ACh-7-nicotinic receptors of those macrophages to inhibit TNF-α. Compared to the HPA axis, CAIP has some unique properties, such as a high rate of neural conductance, which allows immediate modulatory input into the affected inflamed region. Therefore, CAIP plays a crucial role in the intestinal immune response and in homeostasis and presents an extremely interesting target for the development of new treatments for inflammatory diseases related to the intestinal immune system.

The inflammation detection and inflammation suppression functions described above provide the main components of the inflammatory reflex. The appearance of pathogenic organisms activates the innate immune cells that release cytokines. These in turn activate the sensory fibers that ascend into the vagus nerve by synapses in the nucleus tractus solitarius. The increase in efferent signals in the vagus nerve suppresses the peripheral release of cytokines through nicotinic macrophage receptors and CAIP. Therefore, the experimental activation of CAIP by direct electrical stimulation of the efferent vagus nerve inhibits the synthesis of TNF-α in the liver, spleen and heart and attenuates serum concentrations of TNF-α.

CHAPTER 5

THE NEUROCEPTION

The notion of neuroception is central to Stephen Porges' polyvagal theory: continuous evaluation by the autonomous nervous system of the relative safety or danger of a given time or situation and the subsequent release or limitation of the "behavioral repertoire" based on this evaluation.

When we feel confident enough, we record a neuroception by comparing internal and external signals and signals that everything seems to be going well; we are usually able to choose our behavior and the direction of attention. Furthermore, our physiology is able to work in an easy coordination that provides a feeling of well-being.

Our nervous system realizes that we are in danger, whether it is an interpersonal insult or a total attack or simply a change in orientation in gravity, such as during a fall, our free behavior is limited and our attention is aimed at combat or flight type behavior.

When the signal of "threat to life" of neuroception appears, whatever the rational reasons are, our psyche and our body will react with the classic signs of immobilization and freezing as dissociation, physical weakness and fragility or inertia of being.

All these responses are not intentional in their basic organization and, although they can be strengthened through use (ie through conditioning), they are fundamental to their independence and are more fundamental for involuntary processes of our organs.

Neuroception takes place in the primitive parts of the brain, beyond our consciousness. This can be compared to a good watchdog always on guard, allowing us to focus on things other than survival, or sleep well and wake up only when intrusions could compromise our survival. Based on neuroception signals, well-defined neural circuits are activated to support the state of social engagement and user-friendly communication behaviors when we are safe, fight or flight defensive strategies when we are threatened, and stop when we are in grave danger.

Many people have their own neuroceptive experiences when they have reached the "sixth sense" and know that they are in danger or that something is threatening, without knowing how they knew it. A girl from one of my lessons once said, "I can turn my back and know that a boy I don't know is looking at me. I feel his eyes on me before he comes close to me." Even if we don't have a logical explanation, and even if we do not know its neural pathways, neuroception is far from rare.

NEUROCEPTION AND DEFECTIVE SURVIVAL

Neuroception gives us access to information that we do not capture with the conscious part of our mind. When it works properly, it is a true gift and can help us survive. It works faster than the treatment of conscious perceptions.

"I knew something was wrong even before entering the room," how can we collect this kind of information? Sometimes we are faced with a conflict between our neuroception and other thoughts: "I felt that something was wrong, but I still allowed myself to talk".

However, neuroception may be defective and if it does not work as it should, we may find ourselves in a difficult situation. Instead of clearly perceiving what is really there, we are distorting what is happening. Defective neuroception occurs when the neural circuits ranging from perception to behavior do not work properly. A person can react to a safe situation as if it were threatening or dangerous, or react to a dangerous situation as if it were safe.

There can be innumerable reasons for a faulty neuroception. Our perception can be blinded by anger, fear, jealousy or apathy, or we can be trapped in traumatic memory. We can be frozen in a state of shock; we may be hungry and have low blood glucose levels; we can be tired, suffer physically or suffer from an illness.

We can feel perfectly normal and be suddenly triggered by something that reminds us of a traumatic event in our past and respond to that memory as if it were happening in the present. We may not really be threatened, but our nervous system could be blocked in the past, ready to fight or flee at the slightest change in the environment.

Failed neuroception can even come from very positive experiences such as falling in love and forming bonds with the partner. Sometimes we feel that a person's judgment is compromised because they are "blinded by love", so that they are not aware of a potentially destructive situation.

The nervous system must be flexible, allowing the whole body to adapt to the current situation and to support different types of behavior, depending on whether the situation is safe, threatening or dangerous. In the case of chemical interferences (drugs subject to medical prescription, other drugs and alcohol), information comes to us from the environment through our senses, but neural circuits do not process information normally and our physiology does not respond in the appropriate way. Alcohol, for example, changes the way we feel and therefore our behavior. Many drugs - prescription drugs and illicit and recreational drugs - also put us in an abnormal physiological and experiential state.

The following story illustrates a defective neuroception caused by biochemical interference. Three friends, young men of about twenty-five, wandered all day on Mount St. Helens, a functioning volcano in a national park in southwestern Washington State. Although difficult, this climb is suitable for anyone who is in good physical condition and at ease climbing steep terrain. Most climbers make the round trip in seven or twelve hours.

The three friends were well prepared for the excursion. In each of their backpacks they had a map, a compass, a first aid kit and a pocket knife with a set of tools. Everyone had good boots, a climbing helmet to protect themselves from falling rocks, a light sweater, sunscreen and dust masks and glasses in case of falling ash. The sun was reflected in the snow and the volcanic ash could be intense, so they had also taken sunglasses with side screens. They brought food and two liters of water each.

They left early in the morning. The weather forecast predicted a clear, sunny day, and they dressed accordingly. Soon they were very hot from the sun and their efforts. They cleared their heads and took off their sweaty shirts.

Body temperature is regulated by neural feedback mechanisms that work primarily through the hypothalamus, the part of the brain that processes information from essential body temperature sensors. When the body starts to overheat, there are several physiological changes. When the temperature exceeds 37 ° C (98.6 ° F), the nerves in the blood vessels near the surface of the skin cause them to dilate, increasing the volume of blood flowing to the skin. This is called vasodilation and allows more blood to reach the small capillaries of the skin. Up to a third of the body's blood can circulate in the skin and is cooled on the surface of the skin by the surrounding air. Sweating also helps cool the body when its moisture evaporates.

A few hours after the start of the climb, the weather suddenly changed. Clouds formed, the air cooled and it began to snow. The three hikers were cold and wore their sweaters. (They weren't wearing wet shirts.) Unfortunately, this layer of dry clothing didn't provide enough heat quickly enough and they didn't have rain gear. In a few minutes, their sweaters were bathed in cold, wet snow.

The hypothalamus works to conserve heat in the event of a drop in body temperature: autonomic reactions of heat conservation are activated, as well as mechanisms that produce additional heat. A normal cold reaction is the secretion of stress hormones epinephrine (epinephrine), noradrenaline and thyroxine. These cause the muscles to tighten and cause chills. The activity of rapid contractions of trembling muscles produces body heat.

Nerves during a stress response also cause a contraction of the muscle walls of blood vessels, called vasoconstriction. This minimizes heat loss by decreasing the volume of blood circulating from the body's core to the skin, particularly to the hands and feet.

One of the young climbers had taken his usual medicines at the beginning of the day to suppress his chronic stress. One of the effects of this medicine is the lowering stress hormone levels in the blood. As a result, his body could not produce a normal stress response during cold periods. He was not shaking, his blood vessels had not shrunk, his arteries and capillaries were dilated and his skin's blood flow was not reduced to prevent further heat loss.

Because of the drugs, he failed to adapt to changes in his environment and became increasingly cold. Cardiac arrest can occur in extreme hypothermia and eventually his heart stopped. This young hiker did not survive because his body was unable to adapt normally to climate change.

This is an extreme account of how chemicals can interfere with our normal responses to dangerous situations, preventing our bodies from reacting appropriately to protect us.

OTHER CAUSES OF DEFECTIVE NEUROCEPTION

Previously, I described the survival value of the shutdown status. When a lion has its jaw in the throat of an antelope or another prey, its autonomic nervous system usually enters a state of blockade in the face of imminent death and the inability to fight or flee may lose the interest of a predator, which saves the life of its prey.

On the other hand, the personal problems of our complex, modern and civilized human life are generally not so dramatic and generally last more than a few seconds. We may not be physically threatened, but we are often challenged emotionally or mentally. We may need to finish a project on time, solve difficult problems in our relationships with people around us, solve an economic problem or take care of a family member who dies of cancer. We must act - do something or say something - to bring our world back into a state of temporary balance. We can't always sit on a beach, relax and enjoy the surroundings.

Furthermore, unlike many wild animals, humans are usually not released from their traumas once the threat or danger has disappeared. Ideally, we should be able to "restore" our nervous system and start again. But often, the effects of traumatic events persist long after the initial shock. The conscious and unconscious memory can remain in our nervous system for months, years, even the rest of our lives. If we do not get rid of it, we may suffer recurrent inappropriate behavior and permanent physical symptoms of stress and arrest.

Abnormal reactions to certain stimuli may occur because we have had a traumatic experience that involves them. The psychological trigger that causes stress or a stopping reaction can be quite specific. The memory of the event takes place like an unexploded land mine, waiting to be metaphorically trampled by a soldier or perhaps years later by an unsuspecting child. The reaction is triggered because something reminds us, consciously or unconsciously, of everything that has traumatized us previously.

CHAPTER 6

VAGUS NERVE VENTRAL BRANCH TEST

SIMPLE EVALUATION OF FACIAL OBSERVATION

According to Stephen Porges, social commitment requires the ability to look and listen. When you talk to someone, you can feel if they are socially engaged or not as they look at you, how well they feel and how much they understand what you are saying.

You can determine if the person is watching and listening by reading the facial muscles. Does the person look you in the face and stare you in the eye, at least sometimes? Do they have their eyes open? Can they hear and understand what you're saying?

The muscles of the face are organized around the openings of the eyes, nostrils and mouth. (See "Facial Muscles" in the Appendix.) When these flat and round muscles stiffen, they close the skin around the openings. The flat and rectangular muscles adhere to the round muscles and can open them more, allowing more light in the eyes, more odors in the nose and more air in the mouth. When we react emotionally, our facial expression changes when we open or close these openings.

Does the other person have slightly raised eyebrows and eyes are relaxed and open? The flat and round muscle surrounding the eye is called the eye's orbicular. (Orbicularis designates a muscle around a facial opening; oculi means related to the eyes.) By contracting this muscle, we close the opening around the eye, reducing the amount of light in the same way that a shutter in an old reflex camera reduces the amount of light entering the lens onto the film.

We squeeze this muscle to squint when we are exposed to intense light, when we want to reduce visual input, when there is something we don't want to see emotionally or when we want to withdraw from external sensory stimuli and contemplate our thoughts. When we tighten this muscle, we move away from the current visual stimuli, far from the here and now. We can remember past events, view future possibilities or enter a state of meditation.

When the flat, rectangular muscles above and below the orbicular eye are tense, they pull the eye more open, allowing much more light to enter. These muscles stiffen when we find something that opens our eyes. The tension in these flat rectangular muscles is an integral part of the emotional expression of surprise. It improves our sensory contribution and helps us to be more present in what happens around us.

It is interesting to note that when our eyes are more open, we can also listen better: there is a neurological connection between the nerves involved in sight and hearing. During a conference, some people open their eyes a little more to better hear what is being said.

When you make visual contact with another person, look for spontaneous facial expressions in the middle third of the face (between the lower part of the eyes and the upper part of the mouth). The small movements here are an indication of the social commitment (or lack thereof) and the flexibility of their emotional responses.

There are two types of facial expressions: those that we put on display to show another person what we feel and those that occur without our conscious "grimace". We can classify the latter into three types, depending on how long they last.

The first type of unconscious facial expression is the chronic tension model, which is more or less permanent, engraved on our faces with deep wrinkles and indicative of our characteristic emotional state.

The second model of emotional tension is less permanent and expresses our current mood. This pattern of facial tensions remains for a while, while a mood lasts, and is usually enough for someone else to get an idea of how we feel.

In the third type of emotional expression, the facial muscles located in the band between the eyes and the mouth rapidly change the tension, up to several times per second. Usually, we can see these spontaneous micro-expression changes in a child. It is rarer to notice these changes in adults, as we are more stuck in our sense of identity or moods. When these rapid changes are observed, they are too fast for us to read them in a cognitive way to definitively say that facial expression indicates a certain emotion, but the fact that these spontaneous movements are there gives us the feeling that the person is open and without fear.

We can experience these rapid changes in facial expression when two people who feel safe with one another make eye contact, look at each other and allow their feelings to flow without censoring them or trying to control them. This is a reflection of the ideal state of openness, when our facial emotional expressions change as quickly as our thoughts. It is very different from a smile, like when we pose for a photo, where we almost grimace in an attempt to show positive feelings.

Can you see a flow of emotions in another person's face (mercurial facial movements that change quickly and show that he feels happy, satisfied, angry, irritated, scared, anxious, sad or depressed), or that his face is flat and immutable, trapped in an emotional expression? Do you have melodic changes (prosody) in your vocal expression when you talk? Or is your voice flat, with words spoken monotonously?

We tend to think of people as immutable identities. However, your interactions with other people are influenced by your mood, which is influenced by the state of your autonomic nervous system at that time.

People in a state of stress can look at us in a threatening way and their attitude can be aggressive. They may not hear what is being said. They may be inclined to react to a single word, escape control and interrupt us in the middle of a sentence.

We may often need to correct them: "But that's not what I said!"

People with fear will avoid eye contact with us or make eye contact only for a fraction of a second and then look away. Breath can be superficial, raising only the ribs of the upper chest and can hold the breath after inhalation.

People in a depressed state tilt their head forward or let it hang, with a face that is expressionless. They move slowly, indicating a lack of energy.

They have no enthusiasm and don't want to start a conversation. Sometimes, before a depressed person does or says something, he will breathe out or sigh.

EVALUATION OF VAGAL FUNCTION THROUGH HEART RATE VARIABILITY (HRV)

In scientific research on the autonomic nervous system, there is a growing awareness of heart rate variability, which may offer us another way to assess vagus nerve function.

When our nervous system functions optimally and we are socially engaged, there are differences over time between consecutive compromises, there are differences over time between consecutive heart beats, following the natural increase and decrease in heart rate in response to breathing, blood pressure, hormones and emotions. Heart rate variability (HRV) is the measure of these differences. The largest variation in time intervals is designated as high HRV.

HRV can be used as an indicator of general health. It is one of the most promising assessment tools for measuring the activity of the autonomic nervous system.24 When the ventral branch of the vagus nerve is functioning properly, the variability of the heart rate is high. There is a growing amount of related research between HRV and health and longevity.

On the other hand, when there is a reduced level of function in the ventral vagus, the person's autonomic nervous system returns in a state of stress or in a state of dorsal vagal activity, as described in the previous chapter. In this case, the differences in time intervals between heartbeats are minor or non-existent and this is designated as low HRV.

A growing body of scientific studies shows a correlation between low variability in heart rate and various psychological/psychiatric problems. For example, HRV is related to emotional states and has been found to decrease in conditions of acute time pressure, post-traumatic stress, emotional tension and high-state anxiety. People who report increased frequency and duration of daily worries have a lower HRV.

Apparently, low HRV is also related to lack of concentration and motor inhibition, which are symptoms commonly found in children with ADHD. There is also a link between post-traumatic stress disorder and low heart rate variability.

In terms of physical health, a low HRV is assumed to be a less favorable overall health indicator. A variety of adverse health conditions may be associated with lower HRV: obesity, diabetic neuropathy, vagus nerve dorsal branch activity, susceptibility to sudden infant death syndrome (SIDS) and low survival rates in premature babies.

People who suffer from obesity generally have a lower HRV. While we might assume that overweight people eat too much, exercise too little and do not have the motivation to change their behavior, some overweight people follow a diet and almost starve with a small improvement in their weight. Some people who want to lose weight work with a psychologist or hypnotherapist to change their self-image. I can't help speculating: what would happen if your weight loss program included the evaluation of your HRV and the improvement of your nervous system of social commitment for the basic exercise?

Many people with sexual dysfunction seek help from their doctor or the advice of a psychiatrist or psychologist. A recent study sheds light on women's sexual dysfunction, indicating that it may be closely related to their heart rate variability. There are studies that draw a similar conclusion on erectile dysfunction in men, pointing out that "the general imbalance of the autonomic nervous system is one of the causes of erectile dysfunction".

HRV studies have shown that lower HRV was found in people with heart damage and was associated with an increased risk of coronary heart disease. The reduction of HRV also appears to be a predictor of mortality after myocardial infarction (heart attack).

A low HRV is related to early death due to various causes besides heart problems, such as COPD. In the United States in 2014, COPD was the third most common cause of death after heart disease and cancer. Breathing patterns other than normal diaphragmatic breathing indicate lower levels of physical and psychological health and there is a relationship between diaphragmatic breathing and higher levels of heart rate variability. In my clinic, I discovered that patients diagnosed with COPD have very few movements in the respiratory diaphragm and their tests show no ventral vagal activity.

It appears that HRV tests can provide valuable diagnostic information and can serve as a rapid screening tool to assess impaired autonomic nervous system activity.

If scientific research confirms that the state of the autonomic nervous system is a factor in psychological problems, it may be interesting to explore the possibility of improving heart rate variability and the function of the ventral branch of the vagus nerve as a first step in treatment problems, without immediately resorting to traditional psychological interventions or prescription drugs.

THE GLOSSOPHARYNGEAL NERVE AND THE VAGUS NERVE (CRANIAL NERVES IX AND X) AND THEIR DISORDERS

Because these two cranial nerves are intimately connected, they are described here together. The glossopharyngeal nerve has a sensory and motor component. Motor fibers derive from the ambiguous nucleus located in the lateral part of the medulla. Together with the vagus and accessory nerves, they leave the skull through the jugular foramen. They provide the styloopharyngeal muscle whose function is to elevate the pharynx. The autonomic efferent fibers of the glossopharyngeal nerve derive from the inferior salivary nucleus. The preganglionic fibers pass to the otic ganglion through the minor superficial petrous nerve, and the postganglionic fibers pass through the auriculo-temporal branch of the fifth nerve to reach the parotid gland. The nuclei of the sensory fibers of the glossopharyngeal nerve are located in the petroo ganglion which is located inside the petroo bone under the jugular foramen and also the upper ganglion, which is small. The exteroceptive fibers provide the faucial tonsils, the posterior wall of the pharynx, a part of the soft palate and the taste sensations from the posterior third of the tongue.

The vagus: this is the longest of all cranial nerves. The motor fibers derive from the ambiguous nucleus and supply all the muscles of the pharynx, of the soft palate and of the larynx, with the exception of the vein tensor palate and the stylo-pharynx. The parasympathetic fibers derive from the dorsal efferent nucleus and leave the marrow as preganglionic fibers of the craniosacral portion of the autonomic nervous system. These fibers terminate on the ganglia near the viscera they supply from the post-ganglion fibers. They support parasympathetic function. Therefore vagal stimulation produces bradycardia, bronchial constriction, gastric and pancreatic juice secretion and increased peristalsis. The sensory portion of the vagus has its nuclei in the jugular in the ganglion and in the nodose ganglion. The vagus carries sensations from the posterior aspect of the external auditory meatus and adjacent fin and sensation of pain from the duramater that covers the posterior cranial fossa.

Test: it is better to test the ninth and tenth nerve functions together because they are usually affected together. Learn about symptoms such as dysphagia, dysarthria, nasal fluid regurgitation and hoarseness of the voice. The motor part is tested by examining the uvula when the patient is made to open the mouth. Uvula is normally in the midline. In unilateral vagal paralysis, the palatal arch is flattened and lowered ipsilaterally. At phonation, the uvula is deviated from the normal side.

The vomiting reflex or pharyngeal reflex is stimulated by applying a stimulus, such as a tongue depressor or cotton ball, on the psoterioric pharyngeal wall or on the tonsillar region. If the reflex is present, there will be elevation and contraction of the pharyngeal musculature accompanied by tongue retraction. The afferent arc of this reflex is submitted by the glossopharyngeal while the efferent is through the vagus. This reflex is lost in the lesions of the ninth or tenth nerve. Try the general sensations on the posterior pharyngeal wall, on the soft palate and on the faucial tonsils and enjoy the posterior third of the tongue. These are compromised in glossopharyngeal paralysis.

NINTH AND TENTH NERVE FUNCTION DISORDERS

The isolated involvement of both nerves is rare and is usually involved together, often the eleventh and twelfth nerves may also be affected. Glossopharyngeal neuralgia recalls trigeminal neuralgia, but is much less common. It occurs as intense paroxysmal pain that originates in the throat from the tonsillar fossa. It can be associated with bradycardia and in such cases is called vegoglossopharyngeal neuralgia. A trial of phenytoin or carbamazepine is usually effective for pain relief. Brain stem injuries such as motor neuron disease, vascular lesions such as lateral medullary infarction or bulbar poliomyelitis can together influence these nerves resulting in bulbar paralysis. Posterior fossa tumors and basal meningitis may involve these nerves outside the brainstem. Complete bilateral vagal paralysis is incompatible with life. The involvement of recurrent laryngeal nerves, particularly of the left, occurs in thoracic lesions and this produces only hoarseness of the voice without dysphagia.

TEST OF THE PHARYNGEAL BRANCH OF THE NERVE

The ventral vagus nerve has several branches. Below is a test of the function of one of these, called the pharyngeal branch, which innervates the part of the throat immediately behind the nasal cavity and the mouth, above the esophagus and larynx. The nerve fibers of the pharyngeal branch of the vagus go to the soft palate and pharynx. This nerve is involved in swallowing and vocal sounds.

The Greek physician Claudio Galeno was the first writer to describe the pharyngeal branch of the vagus nerve and noted that it provided the function of the motor nerve to the muscles of the larynx, which produce the voice. He learned it by examining a gladiator who had been wounded in the neck and lost his voice; Galen discovered that the pharyngeal branch of his vagus nerve had been cut on the side of the neck. To test the validity of his observations, he conducted an experiment with pigs, whose anatomy is quite similar to humans'. He found that cutting the pharyngeal nerve in pigs would stop their cries.

After trying different ways to test the ventral branch of the vagus nerve, I finally chose the following method by focusing on its pharyngeal branch. It has been described in some of the oldest textbooks on anatomy and physiology and is still taught in medical schools in Denmark. Alain Gehin also taught this test method for testing vagal function by looking at the back of the throat. It has been a great resource in terms of my work with craniosacral therapy.

This test evaluates the movement of one of the muscles innervated by the pharyngeal branch, called the palatal hair lifting muscle. In my experience, I find that the condition of this branch is also a good indicator of the function of other branches of the ventral vagus nerve.

Improving the function of the pharyngeal branch of the vagus nerve improves the function of the respiratory diaphragm. When this test shows a dysfunction of the elevating muscle of the veil of the palate, I generally also observe that the client's breathing is irregular, sometimes fast and not particularly deep. Therefore, after the client has performed the basic exercise and this branch is functional again, I observe that breathing has improved, becoming deeper and slower.

HOW TO EVALUATE THE FUNCTION OF THE PHARYNGEAL VENTRAL BRANCH?

Ask the person to sit comfortably in a chair. Then stand in front of him and ask him to open his mouth so you can see the back of his throat. You will need to see the uvula (the small bulb-shaped structure hanging at the back of the throat) and the soft tissue arches on both sides. Sometimes you can see them sufficiently in normal light; otherwise, you should use a small flashlight. (The torch application on an iPhone is perfect for this).

If the person's tongue is blocking your vision of the uvula and arches, ask them to place one of their fingers on the back of the tongue and push it towards the floor of the mouth. You should be able to see the soft palate more easily. (Doctors use a tongue depressor for this, but this makes some people feel nauseous, and I've never had a client gag with their finger.)

See the Appendix for a series of drawings of the uvula. In "Uvula 2", the arches of the soft palate are raised on both sides by the correct functioning of the veil-lifting palate muscles. Check to see if one side of the uvula rises and the other does not; this indicates a dysfunction of the ventral branch of the vagus nerve on the side that does not raise.

The palatal elevator muscles embedded in the soft tissues, one on each side of the uvula. These muscles are innervated by the motor fibers of the pharyngeal branch of the vagus nerve. When they contract, they raise the arcs of the soft palate. They also stick to the ear tube (Eustachian) between the ears and the throat and pull it during the act of swallowing. This is why the ears sometimes "pop" during swallowing as the air moves into the middle ear cavity and the pressure is equalized.

When we swallow, these muscles must contract, lift the soft palate and allow food to enter the esophagus on the way to the stomach, while preventing food from entering the larynx and lungs. These muscles should contract when someone emits the "ah" sound. A well-trained singer will use this muscle to lift the back of the throat before singing the first note of a sentence.

To test the vagal function, I ask the other person to say "ah-ah-ah-ah" and looking at the arches on both sides of the uvula. These sounds must be percussive and detached: short and brief bursts of sound in rapid succession, and not a long and prolonged "aaaaaaaaahhhh", which does not create the desired effect. If there is good function in the pharyngeal branch of the ventral vagus nerve on the right and left sides, these muscles are stretched symmetrically with a clear impulse when the person emits the sounds "ah-ha-ha-ha-ha", raising the arch soft palate equally on both sides.

If, on the other hand, there is a dysfunction of the pharyngeal branch of the ventral branch of the vagus nerve on one side, the nerve impulses do not innervate the elevating muscle of the soft palate on that side and the arch on the soft palate on that side goes up when the person says "ah".

CHAPTER 7

THE HEALING POWER
OF POLYVAGAL THEORY

Many people focus on the negative consequences of stress and are generally not aware of the problems resulting from chronic activation of the dorsal branch of the vagus nerve. The activity of the dorsal vagus is characterized by lack of physical energy, low blood pressure, fainting, breathing difficulties due to constriction of the respiratory tract in the case of COPD and general chronic pain of muscles and joints, often diagnosed as fibromyalgia.

Before the polyvagal theory, we did not have an adequate physiological model to understand the nature of these common problems. The new understanding of the autonomic nervous system established in the polyvagal theory provides us with a physiological model to understand the neurological factors underlying these dysfunctions. Improving the function of the ventral branch of the vagus nerve opens up new possibilities for treating a myriad of health problems resulting from chronic activation of the sympathetic nervous system or from dorsal-vagal dysfunction.

Stephen Porges explains how our autonomic nervous system affects us mentally, physically and emotionally. He postulated that physiological factors such as the autonomic nervous system and hormone levels play a role in determining our psychological state and, therefore, our behavior. If we want to change our psychological state and our behavioral patterns, or help others change theirs, the solutions could be to initiate changes in the state of the autonomic nervous system.

The implications of Stephen Porges' theory have the potential to develop and implement many new treatments. We may not have to rely so much on antidepressants or other mood enhancers, which are expensive, often do not work as desired and in some cases have serious negative side effects.

This book was written mainly for ordinary people, not necessarily only for health professionals, and for anyone who has not found satisfactory solutions to their health needs within the existing treatment modalities. The book can also be a resource for psychologists, psychiatrists, practical body therapists, doctors and other health professionals who are looking for new ways to make positive changes in their clients. This approach can be used as an alternative or as a complement to other types of treatments.

Many of us have difficulty paying the rising costs of medical care or we want to avoid the negative side effects that can result from drugs. The techniques and exercises in this book are a safe and economical form of self-help. Once you have purchased this book, the treatments are free.

COPD AND HIATAL HERNIA RELIEF

Although many people have heard of COPD (chronic obstructive pulmonary disease) only relatively recently, it is one of the most common non-communicable health problems in the world. COPD is a disease state characterized by chronically poor airflow, shortness of breath and coughing. People with this problem cannot physically exert themselves and find it increasingly difficult to breathe.

Currently it is believed that COPD has many causes, including smoking and exposure to environmental toxins, in reaction to which the body creates an excess of fibers that block the airways in the bronchioles and lungs. It is assumed that this airway blockage is the cause of the individual's breathing difficulties.

It is often tough for people with COPD to continue to work actively and maintain their previous lifestyles, so they often have difficulty planning ahead in terms of financial commitments. They often also have difficulty maintaining levels of activity without work and therefore have a reduced quality of life.

Although steroids and inhalers can temporarily improve breathing, problems can recur as soon as the drugs disappear. And inhalers and steroids often have negative side effects when used for a long period of time, so they are generally only recommended for short-term use. Furthermore, most people with COPD worldwide cannot pay for inhalers and steroids and therefore do not have access to them. The conclusion is that there is no known cure for their condition, which steadily worsens until they succumb to premature death.

COPD usually worsens over time until breathing is so limited that it cannot sustain life. People with COPD, therefore, have a reduced life expectancy. Worldwide, COPD affects millions of people, almost 5% of the population, although the actual prevalence may be higher due to insufficient diagnosis. In 2012, COPD was classified as a third-leading cause of death (after heart disease and cancer), killing over three million people.

How is it possible that, although we spend billions of dollars on medical research each year, we cannot yet successfully cure this generalized disease? Are we searching for answers in the wrong places? So far, no effective treatment for COPD is known.

Perhaps there are solutions that are not based on drugs or surgery.

Doctors and hospitals carry out more elaborate and costly tests than ever, but generally neglect the evaluation of the function of the autonomic nervous system. This is unfortunate, as patients can undergo rapid and inexpensive screening tests of the function of the ventral vagus branch, which affects many other body functions.

Restoration of vagus nerve function is a key element for the successful treatment of COPD.

By making the autonomic nervous system work better, it is possible to help people with a wide range of chronic problems who have not been helped by other treatment modalities, whether allopathic or alternative.

SHOULDER, NECK AND HEAD PAIN: CN XI, TRAPEZIUS AND SCM

Besides being one of the five nerves of "social commitment", the cranial nerve XI (the "accessory spinal nerve") has a special muscular function. It innervates the trapezius and the sternocleidomastoid (SCM), two large muscles of the neck and shoulder. (See "Trapezoid" and "Sternocleidomastoid" in the Appendix.) These are the only skeletal muscles under the face and head that are not innervated by spinal nerves. If one of these two muscles is chronically tense or flaccid, it will respond differently to massage treatment and movement training than any other muscle in the body.

Shoulder problems are among the most common forms of musculoskeletal problems. CN XI dysfunction often causes pain and stiffness in the neck and shoulders, and sometimes it is sufficient to simply improve the function of CN X and CN XI with basic exercise to eliminate pain or limit movement in this area. After training, we could try other ways to treat other problems arising from these muscles; for example, see the self-help treatment for migraine described in the second part. Doing the basic exercise also seems to instantly improve the function of the five nerves necessary for the social participation of most people.

Returning to the trapezius and sternocleidomastoid muscles, we note that CN XI dysfunction and/or lack of adequate tone in the trapezius and SCM muscles are involved in many other health problems besides pain and stiffness of the neck and shoulders. These include migraine headaches, forward head posture, breathing difficulties, chronic activation of the spinal sympathetic chain, chronic vagal dorsal state and shorter life expectancy.

Trapezius and SCM also determine factors in the shape and health of the spine. Moreover, the chronic tension in the sternocleidomastoid muscles on one side can change the shape of the back of the head, leaving it flat on one side due to the constant traction of the muscle in the temporal bones (the skull plates behind the ears).

Turning the head on both sides should be a uniform and well-coordinated movement, without stops or jolts, and without deviating from a smooth curve. The head should be able to rotate ninety degrees or a little more.

People often complain of a reduced range of motion, stiffness or pain in the neck and shoulders when they turn their heads to the side. If the pain or stiffness is on the side opposite the direction in which the head is turned, the shoulder problem is probably the trapezius or the sternocleidomastoid muscle on the side to which you are turning. If the pain is on the same side of the rotation, the problem is not the cranial nerve XI and the trapezius and the SCM, but it is probably due to the elevation of the scapula. In the second part there is a series of exercises called "Salamander Exercises", which improve the neck's ability for lateral movements. In the beginning this exercise can be a little painful, but if we are persistent we can increase the range of motion, improve blood flow to CN XI and improve the function of our trapezius and sternocleidomastoid muscles.

We can improve the function of the cranial nerves and improve the rotation of the head to the right and to the left with basic exercises and salamander exercises. But these may not yet be sufficient to allow total freedom around the head, as many other neck muscles are involved in head movement and the tension in each of them may limit the turn of the head.

If we have neck pain on the same side towards which the head turns, the problem is not the cranial nerve XI, the trapezius and the SCM. Most likely, it comes from another muscle, the lifting shoulder blade ("shoulder lifter"). In these cases, working on the cranial nerve XI and on the trapezius and sternocleidomastoid muscles will probably not eliminate all the pain and stiffness.

Massaging the shoulder blades lifters directly gives relief, but only temporarily: muscle dysfunction returns quickly. Probably the problem is that the muscle is not toned. So if you want a more lasting result, massage the supraspinatus muscle (along the upper part of the scapula) to improve the tone of the shoulder blades.

TRAPEZIUS AND SCM MUSCLES IN ACTION

The cheetah is the fastest mammal on Earth, capable of running at speeds of up to sixty miles per hour. Running at that incredible speed, the cheetah keeps his eyes fixed on the animal he is following. The eleventh cranial nerve allows the cheetah to turn its head and, when it turns, its head follows its body.

An antelope pursued by the cheetah looks for unencumbered areas where it can move away from the cheetah without hitting anything. When your eyes find such space, your head follows the direction of the eyes and then your body follows.

Although not as fast as the cheetah, the antelope has an advantage: if it ran in a straight line, the cheetah could easily catch it, but with its light body and slender legs, the antelope can rotate faster. So to avoid being caught by the cheetah, the antelope zigs and zags. The cheetah cannot do it so quickly. Because it is so agile, therefore, a healthy adult antelope will generally survive being chased by a cheetah. The antelope also has the strength to run for a longer period of time and survive a chasing cheetah.

When a cheetah, a lion, a tiger or another predator chases its prey and fails to bring it down immediately, it is exhausted by the intense effort and takes several hours to regain its strength to try again. Therefore, before fighting, the cheetah spends his time studying the pack of antelopes to choose one who is wounded or old, or a baby hidden in the grass near his mother. Half of all antelope offspring are lost to predators before reaching adulthood.

For both the hunter and the hunted, survival depends in part on turning the head effortlessly, and the main muscles responsible for this are the trapezius and the sternocleidomastoid, both innervated by the cranial nerve XI. Since turning the head is a matter of life and death, it is not surprising that the structure of CN XI is highly developed and complex, for an accurate innervation of the individual fibers of these muscles.

USE OF THE TRAPEZIUS MUSCLES IN A CRAWL

The trapezius is one of the first muscles that humans use as children. When a child lies on his stomach, his first movement is to arch his back and raise his head with the trapezius muscles. So with the head up, the child can turn his head and look around using the sternocleidomastoid muscles.

The next stage in the child's development will be to raise the head high enough to put the arms under the shoulders to support the weight of the upper body. With this, the child will soon be able to get up on all fours. In this position, when the fibers of the upper trapezius are stretched, the neck extends and arches, and raises the head and the face looks forward. To do this, the child tightens all the fibers of the three parts of the trapezius in the same way. The child arches the lower back with the lower trapezius, joins the shoulders to the middle trapezius, lifts the head and tilts it backwards with the upper trapezius. In addition to the trapezius muscle, the head is held and balanced in the vertebrae of the neck, partly due to the action of the semispinal capitis, the largest muscle of the posterior neck. So the sternocleidomastoid muscles can rotate the head quite easily.

In this phase of its development, the child supports its weight on hands and knees and moves in a way very similar to the other four-legged mammals. After a short time, the child can start crawling forward, moving with one arm forward and the other back. This asymmetrical pattern of arm movement during crawling requires the asymmetric use of the trapezius muscles.

With the body resting on four limbs, the arms and thighs are at an angle of ninety degrees to the trunk. While the child pushes down with the arms, there is an equal force that pushes the arm upward into the hollow of the shoulder joint and the proprioceptive nerves in the shoulder joint can inform the brain that the arms and shoulders feel good and are in balance.

CHANGES IN THE USE OF TRAPEZIUS WHEN GOING FROM CRAWLING TO WALKING

Human children bear their weight on all fours when they crawl. Humans have the same physical structure as four-legged animals in terms of the muscles, bones and nerves involved in this movement.

We live in gravity and gravity always pushes us down. When we crawl on all fours, we distribute our weight more or less evenly on our four limbs, which have supported our weight by pushing up on our body. This is a stable structure.

When we stood up, to maintain the balance of the hind legs we had to use our muscles and our bones in a whole new way. Everything has changed in the balance of tensions in our muscular and skeletal systems. Instead of a more or less uniform muscle tone in the muscle fibers, some muscles became chronically stiff and others became inert. Instead of supporting our weight on four supports, we completely balance the upper part of the heavy body in the two spherical joints between the legs and the hips when we are standing, which is more unstable than a four-legged posture.

For decades, standing on hind legs can lead to many problems that four-legged animals do not have. Common to most of us is an increase in head-forward posture (FHP) as we age.

When we crawled for the first time, the trapezius muscle held our head high. The three parts of the trapezius functioned as a single muscle in which all the fibers had approximately the same tension. Some of the muscle fibers worked to push the shoulders back and together to support the upper part of the spine, and other fibers that pulled in other directions worked to lift the head back and up.

But when we got up, parts of the trapezius muscle lost their integrity; They were no longer necessary to bring the shoulders back and tilt the head upwards, as before. Instead of acting as a single muscle, these muscle fibers were organized into three functional units, now seen as the upper, middle and lower trapezius, and these three groups of fibers began to function as separate entities. A part, therefore, could be too tight while another part is under tension. This is reflected in the position of the bones not only of the shoulder but also of the spine.

The spine of a human being has a very different shape from that of a horse, a goat or a giraffe. A four-legged animal bears part of its weight on its front legs, in contrast to a human being whose arms hang freely from the shoulder joint. It is no longer necessary to push the arms towards the shoulder joint.

If we have shoulder pain, we often wonder what we did to create pain: we must have raised something heavy or thrown something, like a baseball, which we were not used to. However, an unrecognized factor in creating imbalances that cause shoulder pain could be the changes that have occurred because we are alone on our legs. And it is not known how the habit of sitting still in a chair for life affects our musculoskeletal structure. Not surprisingly, many physiotherapists report that the most common problems they treat are shoulder problems.

The human spine has weak spots that cause torticollis, back pain and shoulder problems. When we stand up, the relationship between the head and the spine changes with respect to when we were on all fours. To balance our legs, the upper part of the trapeziuiz is no longer positioned to hold the head up and back and the head tends to slide forward.

The central part of the trapezius muscles no longer pulls the shoulder blades toward the spine to form a stable base. Instead, for most of us, our shoulder blades slide down our back, forward and around our sides. Compared to the deep barrel chest of a four-legged animal, the upper part of the chest collapses and the belly is blocked. If an actor assumed this position, it would be to play a character who had lost his sense of self-worth.

When the lower part of the trapezius does not work as it used to when we crawled on all fours, our spinal column is shortened and the head advances. These changes are not due to the increase in muscle tension, but to the general loss of a balanced tone in the three parts of the trapezius muscle that were used to keep the head up against the constant attraction of gravity.

Therefore, to improve the function of the trapezius muscle, we need to improve the tone of the muscle fibers in the three parts of the trapezius by stimulating the nerves to the muscle.

A NEW IMAGE OF CN XI

Turning the head is one of the most important and complex movements of the body. It is one of the first movements a child makes, and we know this movement so well that we generally don't even think about it. Trapezius and SCM muscle control requires coordinated tension and relaxation of many individual muscle fibers and this action depends on a well-functioning CN XI.

Most of the anatomical illustrations of CN XI attempt to show all the branches of this nerve in a single design, but I have personally found that these drawings are confusing. To help you clearly understand the complexity of the structure of CN XI, I asked my illustrator to make some new color drawings that show the three parts of this important cranial nerve. (See the "CN XI" series in the Appendix.) A branch of CN XI comes from the brain stem, this was called "cranial division". Now it is considered part of the vagus nerve, the branch that innervates the pharyngeal muscles.

Another branch, called the "accessory spinal nerve", leaves the spinal cord in the neck just below the skull before going directly to the fibers of the trapezius and sternocleidomastoid muscles. There is another branch of the spinal accessory nerve, composed of nerve branches that leave the spinal cord, intertwine, extend to the skull through the large hole, extend across the floor of the skull, and then exit through the jugular hole at the base of the skull.

Despite their various pathways, all the branches of CN XI work together in a coordinated way to innervate the various parts of the trapezius and sternocleidomastoid muscles.

The CN XI and the ventral vagus (CN X) are closely linked, not only functionally, through their role as two of the five cranial nerves necessary for social engagement, but structurally. A clear connection between the branches of the CN XI and the ventral branch of the vagus nerve can be seen after they have left the skull through the jugular hole: the fibers of the CN XI mix with the fibers of the ventral vagus nerve outside the skull for a few millimeters. In addition to the mixture of their nerve fibers after they leave the jugular hole, both CN XI and the ventral branch of the vagus originate in the ambiguous nucleus, a strip of nerve fibers in the brain stem.

Therefore, it is not surprising that the function/dysfunction of the vagus nerve is directly reflected in the function/dysfunction of CN XI. The test for CN XI provides the same results in terms of the function/malfunction indicative of the tests for the ventral branch of CN X.

HEALTH PROBLEMS RELATED TO THE POSTURE OF THE HEAD

Serious health problems can result from kyphosis or forward head posture (FHP), which is related to the dysfunctional trapezius and the sternocleidomastoid muscles. A head-forward posture is the result of poor posture in general.

As we age, many of us lose the good posture that children enjoy; we may have more difficulty breathing and occasional dizziness worries us. These problems are generally not considered medical problems. Doctors tend to assume that they are a natural part of aging and nothing can be done about it. There is no medicine or operation to help remedy these conditions as such.

The neck has a tendency to yield when we have FHP, which allows our head to advance. Our upper chest collapses, reducing the space for the heart and lungs. The head-forward posture also blocks the action of the muscles responsible for helping to lift the first ribs during inhalation, causing breathing difficulties.

As time goes by and the FHP gets worse, we lose a growing portion of our respiratory capacity. FHP is often found in people with respiratory problems such as asthma and COPD. No wonder they experience general fatigue and low energy levels. Research published in the Journal of the American Geriatric Society also reports that they have an even shorter life expectancy than people who smoke a pack of cigarettes a day and that older patients with FHP have a significantly higher mortality rate.

Could the restrictions on the function of these nerves also contribute to Alzheimer's disease, dementia and senility?

In addition to reducing breathing capacity, the loss of internal space in the chest puts pressure on the heart and fills the blood vessels that come and go from the heart. The FHP also compresses the spaces between the vertebrae of the neck and the upper part of the chest, exerting pressure on the spinal nerves of the neck and on the upper thoracic spine.

Furthermore, the head-forward posture compresses the vertebral arteries that carry blood to the head, decreasing the flow of blood to the face, parts of the brain and the brainstem, where the cranial nerves of social commitment V,

VII, IX , X and XI originate. When this happens, as we can expect, we look pale, we lack spontaneous facial expression and are not socially engaged. If these five cranial nerves do not receive adequate blood circulation, they may not work properly and we are probably in a state of chronic stress or dorsal vagal activity.

Many pains, aches and stiffness develop over time due to impaired posture. "The posture of the head forward causes long-term muscle tension, disc herniations, arthritis and pinched nerves."

Dr. Alf Breig, a neurosurgeon and Nobel Prize winner, said: "The loss of the cervical curve lengthens the spinal cord from 5 to 7 cm and causes disease". The characteristic hardening of the neck in the FHP also hardens the entire spine. According to Dr. Roger Sperry, winner of the Nobel Prize in brain research, "90% of brain stimulation and nutrition is generated by the movement of the spine".

People with kyphosis often have difficulty breathing, slight back pain, tenderness and stiffness in the spine. Emotionally, they can experience apathy and indifference on what is happening, also symptomatic of the vagal dorsal suspension.

Viewed from the side, our ear should be directly above the midline of our shoulder. However, as we age, many of us succumb to a forward head posture and we can see that the ear has moved forward relative to the center of the shoulder. In this case, we usually bend, the upper part of the chest has collapsed and our head is no longer balanced in the neck. The neck muscles must work constantly to prevent the head from tilting further forward.

"Every inch of head-forward posture ... can increase the weight of the head in the spine by an additional ten pounds," according to A. I. Kapandji in The Physiology of the Joints. The head itself weighs about twelve pounds and many of us have our head forward two or three inches.

The man in the head-forward posture photograph came to me complaining of difficulty breathing and general fatigue. His forward posture was not the result of muscular tension, but of flabby trapezius muscles. As mentioned above, FHP often results from dysfunction in the trapezius and sternocleidomastoid muscles; the trapezius lacks sufficient tone, while parts of the SCM are in chronic tension. Therefore, improving the muscle tone of these muscles makes the head more aligned.

Many forms of massage and movement work well in the muscles of the body in general.

SCAR TISSUE CONTRIBUTING TO FHP

Scar tissue is formed after surgery to strengthen the body; in the event that a similar injury occurs in the same place in the future. The patient may know intellectually that this additional scaffolding is not necessary, because it is unlikely that there is another incision in the exact same place, but the connective tissue has no way of knowing.

Although the operation itself may have been necessary or even saved a life, the layers of muscles and fasciae contract and thicken as the incision heals and this hardening in the fascial network extends beyond the local area of the incision to strike the entire body. Every surgical procedure has this negative side effect, which is almost never addressed.

Although there may not be much scar tissue visible on the surface, there may still be a large accumulation of scar tissue in the muscles and connective tissue under the skin, and in the deeper layers of the fascia. Although the operation was performed with the aim of minimizing tissue damage, scars form in the deeper layers.

There should be a small amount of dense fluid between the adjacent layers of muscle and connective tissue which allows them to slide freely from one another. However, during an operation, this liquid sometimes dries out when exposed to air, so that, instead of slipping, the layers begin to stick to each other.

Furthermore, after a surgical incision or any wound, the connective tissue cells produce additional collagen fibers that can attach a layer of muscle or fascia to an adjacent layer. When two layers have grown together, they no longer slide as they used to. Many surgeons take more time and care to ensure that the tissues of each layer are sewn together without involving the tissues of other layers.

Unfortunately, some surgeons do not understand the importance of this and could sew random layers in an attempt to save time and money. The result is that the muscles and connective tissue are much less flexible in that area. Scar tissue feels thicker and stronger and forms not only on the surface but even more deeply in the body. If it is a cesarean section, the scar tissue descends from the surface of the skin to the uterus. If it is in the chest or abdomen, the scar tissue limits the space available for breathing.

The healing after an operation unites everything in a knot; the individual layers dry and unite and movement is limited. As the connective tissue in the front of the body is stretched, it shortens the front of the body and pushes the head forward and down. Therefore, I recommend anyone who has undergone chest or abdominal surgery to look for a masseur who is experienced in releasing tension from scar tissue.

The idea behind the treatment of scar tissue is to work on the restrictions in every single layer of muscle and connective tissue and then release the individual layers from each other so that one layer can slide freely on the adjacent layer. I am always surprise by the amount of improvement that occurs in the range of head and neck movements, flexibility of the spine and general posture after scar tissue is released.

RELIEVING MIGRAINE HEADACHES

Unlike the "cold lungs" (COPD), migraines do not take years away from our life expectancy, but they certainly reduce the quality of our life. There are many affordable drugs for migraines, but these do not always work for everyone. Some drugs are also expensive and most have possible side effects. Many people would rather be free from taking drugs completely.

Of the forty-five million people in the United States who suffer from headaches every year, twenty-eight million suffer from migraines.61 In addition to compromising quality of life, migraines are one of the most expensive health problems in terms of time lost from work . This cost alone in the United States was estimated at $17 billion a year in 2005.

Migraine is Greek for "one side of the head". If the pain is not on one side of the head, I don't consider it a migraine. Migraines, often called tension headaches, vary from moderate to severe and are usually severe, sometimes pulsating, and usually last from two hours to three days. They often occur with symptoms of autonomic dysfunction. They start suddenly and often disappear in the same way. This distinguishes a migraine from other headaches that are sometimes described as "deaf", "on both sides of the head" or "as a tight helmet" or that appear slowly, increase in intensity and gradually end.

Migraines, most times, are accompanied by other symptoms, such as nausea, blurred vision, vomiting, fatigue and hypersensitivity to light, sound, smell and touch. Other accompanying symptoms may include visual distortions (seeing auras) and dizziness. Women may report that their headaches occur at specific point in their monthly cycle.

Biomechanical craniosacral therapy offers specific techniques to release blocks to the eleventh cranial nerve at the point where it leaves the skull. I get the best results in treating migraines by improving the function of CN XI before releasing tension in the muscles with light pressure on the trigger points. The relief of migraines is faster and longer lasting. Most of my clients are surprised to find relief in the first treatment.

If the eleventh cranial nerve does not function properly, the ventral branch of the vagus nerve and the ninth cranial nerve are also usually dysfunctional. The treatment of one of the three nerves immediately improves the function of the other two, so that, in practice, we must not treat each of the three nerves one at a time.

Some authors on the topic of migraines believe that "the underlying causes of migraines are unknown" and not knowing the cause makes them difficult to treat. Other studies show that different psychological conditions can be associated with migraines, including the activity of the dorsal branch of the vagus nerve, anxiety and bipolar disorder.

The improvement in the function of CN X and XI, followed by the release of tension in these muscles through the specific trigger points, generally alleviates the migraine in a few minutes.

CHAPTER 8

SOMATOPSYCHOLOGICAL PROBLEMS

A few decades ago, doctors began to diagnose some health problems as "psychosomatic" (which means that the mind causes problems in the body). However, few psychiatrists and psychologists have studied the opposite: is there a somatopsychological problem in which physiology is thought to influence the mind?

The word psychology derives from ancient Greek and means "study of the mind". Today, defining a problem as "psychological" generally means that a psychologist or psychiatrist first looks for the solution in the mind or in the emotions of his clients, using a verbal approach to therapy.

In this traditional, older definition, the body was not mentioned. When Freud began psychoanalysis to help people with their psychological problems, their treatment modality was 100% verbal. He let people talk without interruption and seemed to listen. There was no dialogue; he didn't even make eye contact or watch his patients face to face. People have remained in psychoanalysis for years, often going to sessions several times a week.

Someone must be a doctor before being trained as a psychiatrist. Then they undergo their psychoanalytic process, which can take several years. At one time there were very few trained psychiatrists and most people could not afford treatment.

Psychologists have created a new picture different from that of classical psychoanalysis. Clinical psychologists are educated for a period of a few years in a university program. To help their patients improve their emotional states and change their behaviors, they rely on various models of the human psyche and interact with their patients using various verbal approaches. They are generally looking for solutions to specific problems. Although not as expensive as years of psychoanalysis, psychological treatment is still expensive and requires the time of a qualified professional in an individual situation.

Some therapists offer group therapy, which is even less expensive, as many patients share the cost of a session. However, this process is more random, since everyone in the group, trained or not, gives their opinion in a session.

Today we are moving further away from these modalities and we rely mainly on prescription drugs to change our behaviors and emotional states. After an initial period of professional consultation to select the drug and the dose, patients can spend long periods of time taking their pills without visiting a health professional. Although prescription drugs can be expensive, they are convenient compared to individual therapeutic processes and ongoing appointments with psychologists or psychiatrists. However, as more and more people take these drugs, this type of treatment involves a growing expense for the individual, as well as for insurance companies and the national economy.

Since psychiatry and psychology started with an exclusive emphasis on the mind and, due to the current availability and widespread use of prescription drugs, we could lose something else that could help with health problems that these types of treatments claim to treat. Perhaps there is something within our reach that has no negative costs or side effects.

In this chapter, we will examine the body to find alternative and complementary solutions to mental and psychological health problems. We will investigate the possibility of regulating our nervous systems and our emotional states and behaviors.

EMOTIONS AND THE AUTONOMIC NERVOUS SYSTEM

Are we open, friendly, communicative and cooperative? Are we closed, depressed or apathetic? Or are we angry, aggressive, anxious, afraid or withdrawn? How do we behave towards other people when we are in these different states?

The way other people respond to us is based on a combination of the state they are in and the state we are in. Our emotions develop in the interaction between the state of our autonomic nervous system and theirs.

As mammals, we are social animals and we need others. We all face challenges and uncertainties from time to time, and to improve our chances of survival and satisfaction, we depend on our interaction with others: family, friends, neighbors, colleagues from work and our social network. The way we feel in a given situation or about a specific person is a factor in our behavior. Does anyone need our help? Do we like sharing time with them? Is it usually supportive? Are we willing to support it? Do we work well together? Do we feel safe? Is there any possibility of cooperation, exchange and friendship?

If we are single and going out with someone, is there a chance of intimacy and a long-term relationship with the other person as a possible partner? If we are married or have an ongoing relationship, do we have enough time together when we are both socially engaged? The more good times we share, the more we have to take advantage of when things get tough.

The correct function of the five cranial nerves of social commitment is essential for our communication and to establish connections with others. These five nerves facilitate our hearing, shape the sounds of our speech and help us understand what others are saying. Can we look at the other person calmly and directly or do we exclude them from our field of vision? If we feel happy and safe, we can usually have a normal two-way conversation, listen to what is being said and look at the other person to exchange meaningful visual cues.

A SELF-REGULATING AUTONOMIC NERVOUS SYSTEM

Social interaction with people who are in a state of balance and social commitment is perhaps the most natural and useful way to achieve self-regulation. If we have a problem, it is often enough to simply talk to a friend. We could sit and eat, or enjoy a cup of coffee or a beer together. We could sing, dance or take a walk together.

Another way to self-regulate our autonomic nervous system is to do the exercises in this book. Many other cultural practices and traditions around the world have been used for centuries with good results: meditation, tai chi and yogic breathing (pranayama), just to name a few. When we meditate, we stand still, overcoming any impulse to fight or run. We also learn to stay awake, avoiding the tendency to withdraw and disassociate ourselves. When we do tai chi, we move slowly, simulating the movements of a very relaxed state. Moving slowly also makes it easier to feel our body and be present in it.

If we can maintain a ventral vagal state, or at least return quickly after stress or emotional withdrawal, we can achieve optimal health and well-being. We can pave the way to realize our human potential, enjoy ourselves with other people and do what we want with our lives.

CHAPTER 9

COMMON PSYCHOLOGICAL DIAGNOSTICS

ANXIETY AND PANIC ATTACKS

Since the beginning of psychiatry in the late nineteenth century, much attention has been paid to anxiety disorders.

Occasional anxiety is a normal part of life. We may feel anxious about a problem at work before taking a test or making an important decision. But anxiety disorders involve more than temporary worry or fear. For some of us, anxiety can become excessive and, although we realize it, we may have difficulty controlling it, so that anxiety can negatively affect our daily lives.

For a person with an anxiety disorder, anxiety does not disappear and can get worse over time. Feelings can interfere with daily activities, such as job performance, school work and relationships. Modern surveys show that some form of anxiety disorder affects up to 18% of people in the United States in a typical twelve-month period; during their lifetime, 30 percent will experience an anxiety disorder.

What we call "fear" is a psychological process that involves activating the nervous system in a threatening situation. Fear can immobilize us (through vagal dorsal activity) or mobilize us to fight or flee (from sympathetic chain activity). Physical symptoms can include rapid heart rate (tachycardia), increased breathing, release of high levels of stress hormones, redness, difficulty speaking and sweating in the palms of the hands, soles of the feet and armpits.

Anxiety is similar to fear in terms of physical manifestations. However, anxiety does not necessarily occur in response to a real situation. Something can remind us of an event in our past, or we can project our imagination into something that could happen in the future. In any case, the threat is not happening now. However, this emotional state is real and exists in the body at the present time.

When we are anxious, we know that we cannot eliminate the worries from our minds. If another person tells us that there is nothing to worry about, it does not silence our minds; sometimes it can disturb us even more. We can answer: "Are you saying that my feelings are not real?"

Panic attacks are short experiences of intense terror and apprehension. They escalate sharply and generally reach their peak in less than ten minutes, although unpleasant feelings can continue for several hours. Sometimes, the specific cause of a panic attack is not obvious. In other cases, we can determine what was caused by general factors such as stress, fear or even excessive exercise.

People who have a panic attack show recognizable signs of fear. Its physical symptoms include tremors, confusion, dizziness, nausea and difficulty breathing. Their appearance seems tense, their skin is pale and they have increased sweating in the palms of the hands, the soles of the feet and the armpits. Their sweat has a characteristic smell.

Dogs and other mammals respond immediately to body odors arising from different emotional states. People also instinctively react to the smell of fear in another person, even if they are not aware of it. Many people try to mask olfactory signs of fear and anxiety by using perfumes, deodorants or foot powder. However, it is difficult to mask a cold and wet hand during a handshake when you meet someone.

Sometimes, anxiety and panic attacks can be effectively addressed with exercises or practical techniques that help us get out of a state of sympathetic nervous system or vagal dorsal activation towards a state of social engagement.

Sometimes we refer to "the drop that made the pitcher overflow". If an anxious person regularly uses the basic exercise, he can minimize the frequency and intensity of panic or anxiety attacks and, in some cases, even prevent attacks. Practicing regularly is like reducing the amount of water in the jar, so it can contain many more drops without overflowing.

It is also important to keep in mind that anxiety can be a side effect of a prescription drug or indicate a substance abuse problem, since drugs and other chemicals alter the state of the autonomic nervous system.

SOCIAL REGULATIONS AND STATES OF ANXIETY

Simple and daily social interactions with family members, friends and colleagues who support it can help regulate our psychological state. We must not underestimate the importance of conversing, and simple social situations such as eating together, drinking coffee or taking a walk with someone. Good social relations help our nervous systems to regulate themselves.

How to eliminate weeds from a garden; if we have been victims we must eliminate or minimize the contact with people who make us feel bad and maximize the time we spend with the people who support us and make us feel better.

When we have been traumatized and then we are socially involved and leave treatment, we will encounter new situations where we may feel threatened again. At the beginning, we may need the support of a therapist to restore a state of social commitment, but the ideal result is having the tools to help us. Whenever we go back, we weaken the control that the traumatic model has had on us; we can rest and restore ourselves, making more energy available to face the next challenges of life.

If we believe that our social network is inadequate, we can also experiment with useful and positive interactions when resorting to health professionals such as masseurs, consultants, trainers, psychologists or psychiatrists. We can choose to consult a teacher or a religious or spiritual leader.

We can also find comfort in prayer or read religious and spiritual texts to help put things in perspective.

DEALING WITH ANXIETY USING YOUR VAGUS NERVE

How often in everyday life do you deal with anxiety?

This section is for you if you find yourself too stressed, stuck in irrational thoughts, or even feeling nauseated, chest pain and heart palpitations.

By naturally stimulating the vagus nerve, you are about to learn a simple but very effective technique to deal with anxiety. This powerful method can be used at any time, anywhere, to relieve stress and anxiety; at home, when traveling, and in those horrible business meetings, of course.

Did you know that the FDA has approved a surgically implanted device that successfully treats depression by regularly stimulating the vagus nerve?

But I hope you don't need an operation. Through following some basic breathing techniques, you will enjoy the benefits of stimulating the vagus nerve.

The vagus nerve is the parasympathetic nervous system's most important element (the one that calms you by regulating the reaction to relaxation).

The vagus nerve acts as a bridge amidst the mind and body, and it's the wiring behind your heart's emotions and instincts. The key to managing your mental state and levels of anxiety is the ability to activate your parasympathetic system's calming nerve pathways.

On request, it is not possible to control this part of the nervous system, but it is possible to indirectly stimulate the vagus nerve by immersing the face in cold water (immersion reflex).

The nerve can also be stimulated by attempting to exhale while holding the mouth closed and pinching the nose. This greatly increases the pressure inside the chest cavity, thereby stimulating the vagus nerve and improving the vagal tone. Singing, and of course diaphragmatic breathing exercises, strengthen this living nervous system, and will pay huge dividends.

Now it's time to put this diaphragmatic breathing technique into use. Breathing with the diaphragm (abdominal breathing) is the basis for proper relief of anxiety.

The diaphragm is the main muscle of the body. It has a bell shape and expands (or flattens) as you inhale, this acts as a piston creating space in your chest cavity so that your lungs can expand and air flows in.

This creates pressure on the abdomen, pushing the organs down and out, thus widening the belly. That's why good breathing practice is described as breathing abdominally or belly breathing.

Breathe with a partially closed glottis in the back of the tongue; the glottis is closed when you hold your breath. We want it to be partially closed here. It's that feeling when you exhale and make a "Hhhhh" sound in your throat to clean your glasses, but without making a sound.

When you're about to sleep, it also feels like the way you breathe when you're about to snore a little.

By controlling the glottis, you are controlling of the air flow during both inhalation and exhalation.

Try it now by practicing this technique of diaphragmatic breathing:

Inhale diaphragmally through the nose, with the glottis partially closed, as if almost emitting a "Hhhh" sound for a count of 7. Hold your breath for a moment. Exhale through the nose (or mouth), with the glottis partially closed, as if almost emitting a "Hhhh" sound for a count of 11. This is one breath cycle; go for 6-12 cycles and observe the results.

Practice, practice, practice. The more you train, the more effective it will be.

Essentially, once your newly acquired breathing capacity is established and abdominal breathing becomes a routine, the body can continuously work at a much lower level of stress.

You will also notice (or sometimes you won't even notice) how your breath responds to stressful situations; your body will be conditioned to control your breathing automatically, resulting in less stress and anxiety.

One of the ways of dealing with anxiety is to learn, through proper breathing, to stimulate the vagus nerve. The vagus nerve serves as a bridge between the mind and the body and regulates the relaxation response. By practicing diaphragmatic breathing with a partially closed glottis, you can stimulate your vagus nerve. Use your downtime to consistently practice this technique; make it a habit, and the results will amaze you.

ANXIETY IN CHILDREN

Parents or other adults often tell children: "There is nothing to fear". In many cases, the tranquility of a loving father or a trusted friend is enough to make someone feel safe.

However, it would be even more effective if the adult had started by saying "I understand you are afraid". This gives the child the certainty of being heard and the awareness that fear (like other emotions) is a normal life experience.

The adult can continue: "There is nothing to fear. Everything will be fine." So, a small hug helps the child to have positive physical contact and can transfer the adult's relaxation.

PHOBIAS

Phobias are the largest category of anxiety disorders and can be disabling. A phobia is characterized by an experience of extreme fear, with a specific trigger that triggers a state of anxiety or a panic attack. Physiologically, fear arises from a reaction in the sympathetic division of the autonomic nervous system.

It is estimated that between 5 and 12 percent of the entire world population suffers from phobic disorders.67 Victims often expect appalling consequences when they encounter the object of their fear. They want to escape, but they are immobilized. They can understand intellectually that their reaction to fear is irrational and disproportionate to the potential danger, but they are still overwhelmed by their fear.

Psychologists and therapists often focus on the object of fear, such as heights (acrophobia), not having enough space (claustrophobia) or spiders (arachnophobia). Their diagnoses focus on triggers, which may or may not be easily linked to specific biographical events. A phobia can be caused by past experiences, for example, when someone encounters a threatening person or a life-threatening situation. A phobia can easily come from a virtual experience, in which the person suffering from the phobia actually did not experience the event; for example, it could be because someone else has told a story or they've seen a scene from a movie.

To better understand something, we tend to classify it and give it a name. But, instead of considering ablutophobia (fear of washing) as substantially different from atrophobia (fear of noise), for example, it may be more useful to divert attention from triggers and towards a useful understanding of physiological activity in the autonomic nervous system in all cases of phobia.

You may be able to help people with phobias if you can help them return from a state of extreme fear to a state of social commitment using the basic exercise (see Part Two). The effect can be similar to what parents do when they help their children by hugging them until the child relaxes and feels safe again.

While physical contact is natural between a parent and a child, there should be no physical contact in a professional psychological intervention. Therefore, a therapist must find another way to make the client feel safe again, and directing him to use the basic exercise could be the ideal solution.

ANTISOCIAL BEHAVIOR AND DOMESTIC VIOLENCE

Most people consider normal human behavior as an expression of positive social values. However, when people are not socially engaged, it is often difficult for others to understand their behavior.

Some people who commit aggressive acts have no idea that there is something wrong with them. They are convinced that the other person has caused or justified their behavior. In other words, aggressive people believe that their actions are a natural response: "He made it happen". They could also consider his action as helping the other person: "It is the only way he will learn".

It can be difficult to understand the reason why normal people commit violent crimes. By observing their actions, we can conclude that they lack empathy, but this does not tell us what is happening within them. What drives them? Is it territory, power, money, sex, jealousy or perhaps alienation? Or is it just an unpleasant feeling that intensifies and then explodes like a bomb in antisocial behavior? Many violent crimes are not premeditated.

CONTINUOUS DOMESTIC VIOLENCE

Domestic violence is very different from facing the enemy in a war or being a victim of casual violence on the street. Some people become victims of domestic violence simply when a loving relationship becomes sour.

We change our approach from the perpetrator to the victim. A man and a woman are attracted to each other and spend more time together; eventually they move in together and start a family. She feels safe with him; she might even think he's her protector. Then, one day, he suddenly loses his composure and hits her. It's a surprise, and she starts to cry.

When things calm down, he hugs her and tells her he's sorry. She asks him to promise that he will never do it again, and he promises it. After a while, they leave the incident behind. At first she is cautious, but seems to have calmed down. Their life together continues as before, almost.

One day, out of nowhere, he gets angry and hits her again. Not only do you have physical pain, but you also feel threatened. When his anger vanishes, he says he regrets it. Once again, they kiss and make up, but while this cycle repeats itself, at a certain point it passes from feeling safe to living in constant fear. He is physically stronger, so she can't win in physical combat. Sometimes she dreams of hitting him with a pan while he sleeps.

She considers taking the children and running away. But where would she go? Where would she live? What would others say? She feels trapped and sees no viable option. Reluctantly, she remains. But the joy she originally felt with him at the beginning of their relationship is dead. She realizes that it has cooled emotionally, which worries her even more: "What's wrong with you?"

After some other incident, she loses the will to defend herself or to escape. She simply resists and dissociates from her body when attacked, as if she didn't care what's happening to her. She can even see herself from afar when she is hit. She just hopes this will end soon. But in the end, she even stops waiting.

This woman made a long, unwanted journey from love (social commitment) to mobilization with fear (fighting and/or escape) to immobilization with fear. She succumbed to a state that we can describe as "Freeze", with the accompanying emotions of apathy, detachment and despair. Perhaps surrendering and being passive when he attacked her helped her survive; he could hurt her even more if she fought or ran away and he followed her.

She is too ashamed to tell other people, so she suffers alone. The answers of others can often seem a condemnation: "If it was so terrible, why didn't you run away?" "Why didn't you call me? I would have helped you." "How could you let him continue to do this to you?" "If you were so stupid and you didn't do anything, it's your fault." No feeling of being understood, no feeling of security and support.

It is unlikely that other people understand that their nervous system has been influenced on an evolutionary scale from social commitment to stress and, finally, to abstinence and apathy. It was her traumatized nervous system that contributed to her behavior. People assumed it was the same person they knew before: a rational person who works well and is socially engaged. People can be quick to judge without understanding the instinctive and emotional mechanisms underlying these changes.

As a first step, an abused woman must find a safe environment in which she is free from further abuse. Past events have already happened and we cannot change them, but we can change the way we react to them emotionally.

CEREBRAL CHANGES OF DOMESTIC VIOLENCE

With traumatized victims and perpetrators, there are real changes in the structure and function of their brains, especially in the amygdala.

The amygdala is found in the temporal lobe, in the midbrain. It is involved in how we respond emotionally to events and information and helps determine how we behave when we face potential risks. In scans, the amygdala shows more activity during negative emotional experiences and when we endure repeated or prolonged periods of stress, our amygdala widens. An enlarged amygdala can make it easier to enter a state of stress or arrest.

The hippocampus is located in the temporal lobes near the amygdala, and this is where we store our non-traumatic memories. When the amygdala widens, the hippocampus contracts due to continuous exposure to dangerous and threatening experiences.

POST-TRAUMATIC STRESS DISORDER (PTSD)

Post-traumatic stress disorder (PTSD), sometimes called post-traumatic stress syndrome (PTSS), has become a common diagnosis. With the wars in Iraq and Afghanistan, we have become increasingly aware of the huge number of veterans affected by post-traumatic stress.

TRAUMA AND THE AUTONOMIC NERVOUS SYSTEM

Ideally, if we have a resilient autonomic nervous system, we recover a state of social commitment after a period of time after a traumatic event. Unfortunately, many people do not recover.

We all experience intense, shocking and distressing events, but we react differently to similar events. Some of us are able to overcome them quickly, return to a state of balance and social commitment and continue with our lives. Others have changed because of what happened and the effects can be lasting, exhausting and even disabling. The negative consequences can also last for the rest of a person's life. If a person is stuck in a state of spinal sympathetic activity, "post-traumatic stress" is an accurate description.

However, after the trauma, not everyone is left in a state of chronic stress. Many people remain in a state of dorsal vagal activity with depressive behavior and describing their conditions as "post-traumatic stress" is inaccurate, confusing and leads to ineffective treatments. It will be more accurate to talk about two different outcomes after the trauma: a state of chronic activation of the spine, a post-traumatic sympathetic activation (the response to the fight or flight stress) or a post-traumatic state of chronic vagal dorsal activity (suspension or arrest).

Sometimes, a person with post-traumatic stress disorder switches between these two states, avoiding a state of social commitment. The problem for many soldiers returning home with a diagnosis of post-traumatic stress is that often the people who treat them have not found effective treatments. Unfortunately, many men and women who have served their country in battle, therefore, end up socially isolated and an alarmingly high number of them commit suicide.

We get a clearer and more useful image by differentiating between post-traumatic stress and post-traumatic arrest. Are the patient's behaviors and symptoms a sign of sympathetic activity in the nervous system or dorsal branch activity? The activity of the sympathetic chain produces what we generally describe as stress behaviors, while dorsal vagal activity leaves a person withdrawn and shows a depressive behavior. Stopping in any degree is caused by an increase in activity in the vagus dorsal (old) branch. Mammals share this reaction with almost all vertebrates up the evolutionary scale, to fish without jaws like lampreys.

In the treatment of post-traumatic stress, therapists tend to focus on the trauma itself rather than on the psychophysiological fixation that followed the event. Remembering the experience and telling someone else is undoubtedly a way to relieve post-traumatic stress, but it is not the only way and it can often be counterproductive, since the person can be traumatized again by telling it. In a lot of cases, it is easier and more effective for a therapist to avoid the memory of the event and work with practical exercises or treatments to restore a state of social commitment.

ACTIVITY OF THE DORSAL BRANCH AND PTSD

The goal of my treatments for people diagnosed with PTSD is to get them out of a state of activity in their sympathetic spinal circuit or dorsal vagal nerve and bring them to a state of social commitment. The next challenge is to help them stay socially involved by repeating this when necessary.

It is not correct to suppose that the activity of the dorsal branch is a purely psychological problem that must be treated verbally; a psychophysiological state is often a more appropriate way. Physicians often biochemically treat the mental manifestations of dorsal branch activity with antidepressant drugs, many of which function as stimulants and create an excited state in the nervous system. This helps people to mobilize in general, but does not produce desirable social behavior or states of happiness or joy.

A new understanding of stress and the role of vagus nerve branches can be of great help in the treatment of many psychiatric and psychological disorders. The physiological states driven by the activation of the visceral organs through the vagal dorsal branch cause an enormous loss of resources and loss of quality of life, not only for individuals, their families and the people around them, but through its economic impact on society in the treatment of these psychological problems.

RESTORATION OF FUNCTION AFTER A TRAUMATIC EVENT

The autonomic nervous system usually has an intrinsic capacity to regulate itself. If we feel safe both in our environment and in our body, it is natural to be socially engaged, share and be at ease with others. Similarly, we can be immobilized without fear of resting, rebuilding the body and restoring ourselves.

Social interaction with other people in whom we feel safe often restores our ability to return to stress or close to social commitment. However, this does not always happen. The current situation could be over; we have stopped running or fighting, and now we are free from threats or dangers, but our nervous system could remain stuck in the past and remain in a state of struggle, flight or freezing (dissociation).

Post-traumatic stress occurs when the fight, flight or freeze responses are awakened but not completely discharged.

When our nervous system is liberalized, we dissociate ourselves. We lose contact with our body, with other people or with the here and now. Therefore, we become ineffective and vulnerable. Many common phrases describe it; "Out of the world", "not with it", "outside of myself". In terms of the nervous system, we have lost function in the ventral branch of the vagus nerve.

The trick to restoring the vagal self-regulating function is to do something to return to Earth, return to our senses, be in our body and return to the here and now. Some of us are helped by meditation, some pray, others go fishing or move to a quiet place just to reflect.

Some of us may ask for the help of a therapist, a coach or a teacher. The important thing is not what these health professionals call their method, or what positive results they claim to offer, but whether their methods really work for us or not.

If we are trying to restore the regulation of our nervous system through social interaction, we need to make sure that the people we choose to interact with work well. A simple way to evaluate this is to ask ourselves: "When I am with them, do I feel better afterwards?" We have all had experiences of being with people and feeling worse.

Once we are balanced and self-regulating again, we should find that we have greater resilience when we are with the same people who brought us down before. Ideally, we will be less affected, or at least we will recover more quickly. Although sometimes we can reduce the amount of time we spend with people who are bothering us, we can't always avoid them, so it's useful to be able to respond more resiliently.

It is also important to be patient. Helping us successfully, even once, will make it easier next time. Being alive implies facing a constant succession of challenges, threats and dangers, and regulation is an ongoing process to successfully face difficulty when it presents itself. It will be much easier for us to face a new challenge if we can stay on the ground, not to disturb and maintain or quickly recover a well-functioning ventral branch of the vagus nerve.

DEPRESSION AND THE AUTONOMIC NERVOUS SYSTEM

Depression remains the leading cause of medical disability in the United States and Canada, accounting for nearly 10 percent of all medical disabilities. In recent years, doctors have prescribed more and more antidepressants.

People with a diagnosis of depression, or people in a depressed state, generally lose interest in activities that were once fun. They experience loss of appetite, overeating or other digestive problems. They have reduced energy and become inactive, introverted, apathetic, defenseless and asocial. They can feel sad, anxious, empty, hopeless, worthless, guilty, irritable, embarrassed or restless. They can experience lethargy, lack of energy and lack of goal-oriented activity. They may have difficulty concentrating, remembering details or making decisions and are often affected by the pain and discomfort of fibromyalgia. They can contemplate, try or really commit suicide. All of these can be symptoms of activity in the dorsal branch of the vagus nerve.

If we consult with a doctor because we do not feel well, the doctor can ask questions and determine from our answers that we are depressed or stressed. Instead of considering the possibility that the condition is transient, the doctor assumes that it is semi-permanent and we are given a drug. There is often a dose adjustment period until we feel better. So we can continue taking the medicine for months or even years.

Many people who come to me want to stop taking their medications. Although I support you in this desire, I tell you to do it only in consultation with the doctor who prescribed it. Furthermore, I recommend searching the Internet for information on the negative side effects of the drug and discovering all available information on withdrawal symptoms that could occur if you stop treatment.

A study published in the Journal of the American Medical Association showed that antidepressant prescriptions do not work better than placebos in mild cases of depression. It is known that these drugs often have negative side effects. However, antidepressants continue to be the most consumed type of drug in the United States, with 270 million prescriptions written for them each year.

This raises some obvious questions: why do doctors prescribe so many antidepressants? Could we benefit from adopting a new approach? I believe the basic problem is the lack of understanding of the nature of the autonomic nervous system, which should normally be flexible, resistant and only temporarily influenced by stress factors. Polyvagal theory can show the way to this new approach.

The medical literature has generally focused on the physiology of chronic stress, with less attention to the physiology underlying depression. When people come to my clinic with a diagnosis of depression from a psychologist or psychiatrist, or when they show depressive behavior, I find that their problem is usually accompanied by a state of activity in the dorsal branch of the vagus nerve.

Before the polyvagal theory, vagal dorsal problems lacked a physiological model in terms of the nervous system, and perhaps this is why it was so difficult to find safe and effective treatments without drugs for conditions like depression. Stephen Porges' polyvagal theory focuses on the relationships of the autonomic nervous system, emotions and our behavior, and his work has attracted a growing interest in the application of these understandings by psychologists, psychiatrists and a variety of talented trauma therapists.

BIPOLAR DISORDER

Bipolar disorder is a pattern of behavior characterized by periods of high activity and euphoria ("mania"), which alternate with periods of depressive behavior.

The mania is characterized by abnormally high energy levels and a euphoric, exultant mood. The periods of mania are followed by periods of activity of the dorsal branch of the vagus nerve, experienced as low energy. In some people, these mood swings are separated by periods of "normal" feelings; in other individuals, the states of activity of the dorsal branch and the mania alternate without respite. These people often dissociate from feeling their own bodies and may suffer from psychotic symptoms such as delusions and hallucinations. Bipolar problems affect up to 4 percent of the American population.

From the point of view of the polyvagal theory, the manic phase can be seen as the activation of the spinal sympathetic chain. In a manic state, the person spends large amounts of energy and performs many actions without necessarily rejoicing or being satisfied with them.

CHAPTER 10

AUTISM SPECTRUM DISORDERS

The term autism spectrum disorder (ASD) comprises autism, Asperger's syndrome and other conditions. (ADHD is not defined as an autism spectrum disorder). ASD covers a wide range of symptoms, and levels of disability that can occur in children or adults. These symptoms, which could be brain development disorders, can cause significant social, behavioral and communication challenges. However, there are no neuronal tests for these disorders.

There are many different categories of autism. Disorders affect every person in a unique way and range from very mild to severe. People with autism spectrum disorders share some of the same symptoms and seem to handle information in their brains differently than other people. The exact causes of autism spectrum disorders are not known. Research has suggested that both genes and the environment play important roles.

The evidence indicating genes is based in part on the observation that if an identical twin is autistic, the other twin is also likely to be. However, despite spending hundreds of millions of dollars, researchers have not yet identified which genes may be defective in autism cases. Ideally, this will be determined soon, but at the moment there is no promising cure for autism spectrum disorder based on genetic research.

Autism spectrum diagnoses are mainly based on behavioral observations by psychologists. However, people who perform the tests generally do not consider the physiological signs of the social commitment portion of the autonomic nervous system. But the autonomic nervous system partly determines the emotional state, and the emotional state is a factor that contributes to determine the behavior. I think if we change a person's emotional state, we can change his behavior.

Can some cases of autism spectrum disorder be interpreted as manifestations of an autonomic nervous system disorder? These people are often in a chronic state of fight or flight or dorsal vagal abstinence. Sometimes, for no apparent reason, they suddenly change from one of these states to another, taking caregivers off guard. Their behavior is often unpredictable and inappropriate for the situation.

Based on my clinical experience, I suggest that autism spectrum tests should include evaluation of the function of the ventral vagus nerve. If it shows dysfunction, further investigations could determine whether bringing the patient to a state of social commitment by optimizing the function of this nerve produces positive changes in his behavior. I think this would be the case.

HOW PREVALENT IS AUTISM?

There is a growing number of people being diagnosed with autism spectrum disorders making this the fastest growing developmental disability, with an annual increase of 10-17% in the United States. About one in sixty-eight children has been identified with ASD, according to estimates by the CDC's developmental disability and autism monitoring network (ADDM). According to other estimates, autism spectrum disorders affect one in ninety children.

The economic costs of autism are also enormous, not only for individual families but also for society as a whole, as requests for medical care and other services related to autism increase.

More importantly, there is also a human loss to our society. Among the personal costs of autism is the high emotional cost required by parents, which cannot be calculated in dollars. Before the child was born, the parents had dreams and hopes of having a family like other families, with well-functioning children. Often, autistic individuals cannot maintain a job and contribute to the workforce, or they may have difficulty raising the next generation. Whatever their goals were before, the family must now prioritize taking care of their child in a new way.

AUTISM AND THE AUTONOMIC NERVOUS SYSTEM

Spinal sympathetic chain activity and/or dorsal vagal activity may be physiological features of the nervous system of people with various diagnoses on the autistic spectrum. They may also have a physical problem resulting from dysfunction in their organs.

Family members or health care professionals may notice that people with autism sometimes react with fear and panic, even for no apparent reason. They can be hypersensitive, react to a stimulus in the environment that other people don't notice, or something that reminds them of something about their past, or they can simply imagine something dangerous. Other people who observe their behavior objectively find that these reactions are unfounded and feel that there is nothing to worry about.

Sometimes people on the autistic spectrum are trapped in states of struggle and flight or closure, or change between these two states. They can be in a closed state, bent and apathetic at one moment, and suddenly extroverted, frightened or aggressive in the next. For others who do not understand their behavior, they react in apparently strange and unpredictable ways that often make them seem unsociable in their behavior. Many parents or caregivers are confused and surprised by these sudden changes in behavior because they are not aware of anything that can cause emotional changes.

Psychological tests for autism evaluate behavior and define different types of autism, but do not consider the underlying physiological factors in terms of Porges' new interpretation of autonomic nervous system function. As a result, the treatments focus mainly on parental training to try to adapt their behavior to the special needs of their children, rather than improving the child's condition so that they do not have these special needs.

The polyvagal theory presents a new bio-behavioral model that links autistic behavior with specific physiological states of the autonomic nervous system. This gives us the opportunity to develop more effective strategies to treat autism.

When we see that many of these individuals are affected by their spinal sympathetic chain or dorsal vagal activity, or hesitate between the two, we can simply say that they are not socially involved. We can therefore concentrate on the use or development of interventions that help them participate socially and improve the function of the ventral branch of the vagus nerve and the other four associated cranial nerves, resulting in greater social behavior.

Stephen Porges chose to work with autistic children and managed to improve the behavior of many of them. He interpreted this as a verification that there was some validity in the model of the nervous system presented in the polyvagal theory. His work inspired me and I also treated autistic people with some success.

HOPE FOR AUTISM: THE PROTOCOL OF THE LISTENING PROJECT

Stephen Porges made important distinctions in his polyvagal theory and listening project that indicate specialized functions of the cranial nerves that go to the muscles of the middle ear and how correct listening allows social engagement. Porges has made a breakthrough in our understanding of hearing, one of the problems that affects about 60% of autistic children.

He described how the problems associated with listening and processing of human voices could be related to the poor function of the cranial nerves V and VII, rather than to the cranial nerve VIII, as in typical deafness, and how the mechanisms involved in listening can be an important part of autism symptomatology.

People on the autistic spectrum pose a challenge in many ways to parents, teachers and other health professionals. Anyone who works with autistic children realizes that they often do not seem to be able to understand what other people are saying and cannot maintain normal two-way communication. Many people on the autistic spectrum do not seem to understand the meaning of what is being said to them and many of them do not speak at all. This is particularly challenging for psychologists and psychiatrists because autistic people generally have difficulty communicating verbally, so word-based therapies are not useful.

Therefore, as usual, your cranial nerve VIII (auditory nerve), which has deep sensory fibers in the inner ear, is tested to determine if the hearing is sufficient. Most people on the autism spectrum pass the standard hearing test, which is usually administered in a quiet room with no background noise or with the subject wearing headphones that eliminate all sounds other than the tested frequencies.

The problem with this test for individuals on the autistic spectrum is that it only measures a part of the auditory mechanism. Stephen Porges realized that in order to hear and understand what is said, people need two other cranial nerves: the trigeminal nerve (cranial nerve V) and the facial nerve (cranial nerve VII).

To learn to speak, we must first be able to listen and understand the spoken language. Porges has discovered that many people on the autism spectrum have a dysfunction in cranial nerves V and VII, which interferes with their ability to listen and understand the spoken language. These nerves originate in the brain stem and each has different branches with different functions, two of which go to two muscles of the middle ear. CN VII goes to the stapedium, a small muscle in the middle ear, and the CN V goes to the tympanic tensor, in the eardrum.

One of the many functions of the cranial nerve CN VII is the innervation of the stapedium muscle. When stapedius works properly, it helps to reduce the volume of sounds that are above and below the frequency range of the human female voice, to help a child focus on the sounds in the frequency range of a mother's voice. When this muscle works properly, a child can easily hear his mother's voice above the background noise, learn his mother's language and communicate with her and other people.

CN VII, which innervates the stapedium muscle, also has other branches, one of which controls the facial muscles (which have been called "emotional expression organs"). When this nerve is not functioning properly, there is often a lack of facial expression. A characteristic of children and adults diagnosed with autism is the lack of natural facial expression. The flat expression on their face makes it difficult for people to read their emotions in a conversation. For this reason, other people tend to think that the autistic individual lacks empathy.

There is a neurological connection between adequate hearing and the muscles that open the eyes. The seventh cranial nerve innervates the flat ring muscle around the eye and people with hearing problems often have drooping eyelids. Raising eyebrows, the way we do it when we listen to something that is a "revelation", can help us understand the spoken language. All these factors underline the importance of listening to the correct functioning of the seventh cranial nerve.

A branch of CN V regulates the tension in the tensor muscle of the eardrum, which participates in the regulation of the Eustachian tube that connects to the throat. The tympanic tensor is similar to the stapedius, which regulates the stiffness of the ossicles (small bones of the middle ear). Stretching the ossicular chain increases the tension of the eardrum, decreasing the volume of low frequency background sounds.

One of the functions of the stapedius and tensor ear drum muscles is to cushion the sounds produced by chewing. If the muscles of the middle ear do not contract sufficiently, the perceived volume of low-frequency sounds can be extremely high and even mask the sounds of the human voice. This condition is called hyperacusis. For people with this condition, incoming sounds can be annoying or even painful. Some autistic children put their fingers in their ears to block out sounds, especially low-frequency ones.

In this condition, a child processes acoustic information only within a limited frequency range, so that sounds in the frequency range of human speech can be lost in the background sounds, while lower tone sounds can be functionally amplified. Children with hypersensitivity to sound can overreact to other people's voices, particularly the low voices of some men. And when you put your fingers in your ears, this can be misunderstood to indicate that your child does not want to hear what is being said, when in reality they are just trying to protect their ears from a painful experience.

Daily noises that include low frequencies (e.g. vacuum cleaners, traffic or escalators) seem unbearably noisy for people with this condition. They can't understand what they are told because of the background noises that annoy them tremendously, even if the same noises do not disturb other people.

One of my patients, an eleven-year-old boy, put his fingers in his ears to reduce the noise every time a train passed some distance from my office window. I had never noticed the sound of passing trains before and my other clients never seemed to react.

A different type of muscular and nervous dysfunction can cause an opposite type of problem in hearing and understanding what is being said. Muscle tone may be insufficient to amplify the sound properly, so not enough sound passes and the child may seem deaf to what is being said. This is often misunderstood as a lack of interest in communication and social activity, or it is understood that the child does not want to respond or do what is required.

Sometimes, children with these problems can become very adept at reading lips and interpreting body language. It may seem that they can have a conversation and be sociable, but they have a problem if the person who is talking is not directly in front of them, so they cannot read their lips.

Some adults also have difficulty understanding what is being said unless they can see the other person's face. People who read lips fix their eyes on the other person's mouth, unlike a person with normal hearing who looks into the other person's eyes or looks away while listening. Adults who have difficulty understanding if more than one person speaks at the same time can avoid going to parties or restaurants full of people, preferring to meet people one by one. Or they can use another strategy: talk all the time to avoid revealing that they can't understand others.

Children on the autistic spectrum may have great difficulty functioning normally in a noisy class. When a child is too sensitive to sound, a high level of background noise can be painful, while children with a functioning inner ear usually find the same level of noise acceptable.

For a child with severe hyperacusis, environmental sounds cause epidemics of pain to those who cannot escape. Going through the different soundscapes of everyday life may seem like the experience of rats in a cage stressed by electric shocks at unpredictable time intervals. Children most times do may not even realize they have a problem. If they are born with hyperacusis, they may not know that their casual traumatic experience is not normal.

Imagine watching a movie with a strong soundtrack: the actors' voices shout at you and you can't wait to get out of the cinema. You leave, holding your ears. But what would happen if you were an autistic child who can't leave the cinema?

In order to study the implications of cranial nerve dysfunction and ultimately to demonstrate the validity of the polyvagal theory, Stephen Porges designed his listening project protocol for a research program conducted with subjects on the autism spectrum.

In a peer-reviewed research, he describes his empirical studies using the protocol of the listening project with autistic children. Porges' research and scientific articles over the past twenty years have opened up new avenues in the treatment of autistic conditions. The identification of a physiological model that may be partly responsible for autistic behavior patterns is a significant advance in our understanding of autism and has opened up possibilities for new forms of treatment. The method he developed has already helped many people improve their communication and social behavior skills.

Porges hypothesized that the reason many children on the autism spectrum have difficulty using language to interact is dysfunction in the neural regulation of the middle ear muscles, as described above. CN V and CN VII, two of the cranial nerves needed for social engagement, originate in the brain stem and have branches that go to those two muscles in the middle ear.

Porges treated a large group of children diagnosed with autism through an ingenious therapeutic intervention. In the investigation of the Protocol of the Porges Listening Project, all the children evaluated had diagnosis on the autistic spectrum and many of them also had hyperacusis. All the children, after receiving numerous hearing tests, received five sessions of forty-five minutes a day for five days.

In one publication, Porges and his group demonstrated that computer-modified music improved auditory processing capabilities and increased vagal regulation of the heart.

A second publication describes two tests conducted by the Porges team. A trial compared a group of children who used headphones only with another group that received computer-altered music, processed with an algorithm to improve the acoustic characteristics of prosody. In the second test, one group received altered music from the computer and the other group received the same music, but without modification. In both tests, only the group that received computer altered music showed a reduction in auditory hypersensitivity.

THE ROLE OF HEARING IN AUTISM SPECTRUM DISORDERS

To be sociable and maintain a two-way communication, people must listen and interpret the meaning of the words spoken by others. As described above, hearing and comprehension problems characterize many people on the autism spectrum. This phenomenon is well recognized. Stephen Porges initially pointed this out in his presentation of the polyvagal theory, and I confirmed it in my practice. However, these hearing problems are often linked to a dysfunctional CN V and CN VII (as Porges discovered) and not to a CN VIII, the auditory nerve, which is often mistakenly held to be the only one responsible for hearing.

When an autistic, Asperger or challenging child arrives at my clinic, I ask the parents to listen to their children. Invariably, they say that your child's hearing was assessed by a specialist ear who reported that it was normal. Most autistic children are tested for hearing in the usual way: they wear headphones and respond when they hear the various volumes and frequencies of the headphone sound.

Parents are almost always told that their child has good hearing, but this loses the core of the autistic child's hearing problem. This is not the child who hears unique tones in a test, without background noise. The question should be: can the child hear the human voice in the presence of background noise? Does the child have the ability to filter background sounds, especially low frequency sounds?

TREAT THE HEARING IN AUTISTIC CHILDREN

A common characteristic of people participating socially is that they generally have a melodic voice and can communicate feelings. This vocal melody, or prosody, facilitates the understanding of other people. In contrast, people with autism often have a flat, monotonous voice, which may seem mechanical and robotic.

Perhaps the reason they lack prosody in their voice is that they can't hear it in other people's voices because of a dysfunctional CN VII. If a child cannot listen and appreciate or hear the emotions communicated by the melody in the voices of others, he cannot understand the benefits of using the melody with his own voice, much less learning to express it.

This voice quality is not primarily a vocal problem, per se. As soon as we help people in the autistic spectrum in a state of social engagement through improved function of their cranial nerves, the quality of their voice changes; they immediately have more prosody and it is easier for others to understand what they say.

Sometimes, hearing can be improved with basic exercise by increasing blood flow to the brainstem, where cranial nerves V and VII originate. The basic exercise can also loosen the tension between the base of the skull (where is located the nucleus CN V) and the first three vertebrae. The neurofasciale release technique can also be sufficient to restore the function of these nerves and improve social behavior.

With the understanding gained from the study of the polyvagal theory, I developed my approach to autism spectrum disorders. I evaluate the function of the cranial nerves V, VII, IX, X and XI, so I use a selection of specific cranial biomechanical techniques to release the restrictions and allow these nerves to function correctly.

Based on the experiences and clinical comments, you can confirm that it is possible to improve communication skills of some people diagnosed with autism.

AUTISTIC TREATMENT

Over the years, I have successfully helped many children and young people with a diagnosis in the autism spectrum. Many of these children have problems with normal social behavior; they don't seem interested in others, avoiding looking at them or looking them in the eye. They seem devoid of empathy and prefer to spend time alone or playing on their electronic devices.

Their parents can designate other young people as "friends" if they can sit together in the same room for periods of time. However, children do not really interact with these friends, but instead sit in their worlds, playing together, but alone.

Some autistic people lack verbal communication skills and cannot participate in a meaningful two-way conversation. They do not seem able to listen or understand what is being said and are not playful. Some do not speak at all; others, when they speak, can repeat what someone else has just said as a parrot or repeat the phrases of a film. Sometimes they continue to talk without stopping because the other person answers.

To start making sense of all the various behaviors exhibited by individuals on the autistic spectrum, I observed that these individuals are not socially involved and have a defective neuroception. I was able to assist some of them by bringing them into a state of social commitment. In several cases, I achieved normal vagal function and improved the function of the other four cranial nerves involved in social engagement. This removed individuals from states of stress or dorsal vagal withdrawal and spontaneously improved their communication skills.

Perhaps one of my most unexpected discoveries when performing body therapy is to find tension in the right sternocleidomastoid muscle (SCM) and a consequent deformation of the skull called "flat back of the head" or plagiocephaly, in every client diagnosed with ADHD or diagnosis on the autistic spectrum. Research published in the journal Pediatrics has reported that this deformation of the skull, usually only on one side, is present in a higher percentage of children with autism and ADHD, compared to children who function normally.

The sternocleidomastoid muscle joins the base of the temporal bone on the side of the skull, so that chronic tension in the SCM muscle significantly deforms the shape of the skull in a particular way. Although this group of clients consists mainly of children and young people, this deformation of the skull is not limited to children; I also see it in many adults who have had difficulty participating socially. This same approach can achieve similar improvements in adults.

Do some characteristic forms of the skull exert pressure on certain blood vessels or nerves within the skull?

The skull of a child is composed of several plates, connected by a resistant connective tissue. A constant pull of the temporal bone due to chronic tension in the SCM muscle can deform the child's skull. If the tension is not released into the muscle, the skull remains out of shape while the child matures.

PART TWO

CHAPTER 11

HOW TO RESTORE SOCIAL COMMITMENT

The second part explores the healing power of the vagus nerve. Optimal health is only possible when we have a ventral branch that works well for the vagus nerve. The exercises and techniques in this part should help most people move from a state of chronic activity of the spinal sympathetic chain (stress) or vagal dorsal activity (arrest) to a state of social commitment. These exercises can also be used to prevent the development of problems in the autonomic nervous system and to maintain a general level of well-being.

When you start doing these exercises for the first time, we suggest you start a simple diary. Write down any symptoms or problems that disturb you. Also, take a look at the numerous symptoms listed in the "Capi Hydra" list at the beginning of the first part. You may want to add one or more of these to your list.

Consider how often a given symptom has appeared. For example, the symptom may occur "all the time", "every morning", "once a week" or "once a month". If you have a headache every day, your goal is undoubtedly to free yourself completely from migraines; however, any improvement would be a positive result.

Also, keep in mind how strong your symptoms are. You can write that "They annoy me, but I still function in the day", "They require me to take medicine", "They are so strong that I can't go to work or participate in normal social activities", "I can't sleep" or "I can't to get out of bed in the morning." You may prefer to evaluate pain or symptoms using a scale of one to ten.

After performing the exercises, you can check the list and observe any changes, for example "Migraines are less frequent", "Pain is less intense" or "I spend less money on painkillers every month". Focus on how the exercises have helped: that you do not have the symptoms so often or that the problem is not so serious. Perhaps the remaining symptoms will diminish or disappear as you continue to do the exercises.

Do you also notice other positive changes, for example, sleeping better? Breathing better? Is your appetite more normal? All this helps to improve health and endurance.

THE BASIC EXERCISE

The objective of this exercise is to improve social commitment. Reposition the atlas (C1, the first cervical / cervical vertebra) and the axis (C2) and increase the mobility of the neck and the entire spine. (See "Axis" and "Atlas" in the Appendix.) And also increases blood flow to the brainstem, where the five cranial nerves necessary for social engagement originate. This can have a positive effect on the ventral branch of the vagus nerve (CN X), as well as on the cranial nerves V, VII, IX and XI.

The basic exercise is effective, easy to learn, easy to do and takes less than two minutes to complete. I usually teach this to my clients in their first session.

BEFORE AND AFTER THE BASIC EXERCISE

Evaluate the relative freedom of movement of the head and neck. Turn your head to the right side as far as you can comfortably. Then go back to the center, take a break and turn your head to the left. How far do you turn on each side? Is there pain or stiffness?

After training, perform these same movements again. Is there any improvement in the range of your movements? If there was pain during head rotation, did the exercise reduce the level of pain?

Most of the people I have treated are surprised to experience an improvement in the range of motion by turning the head left and right. Improved movement of the neck often accompanies an improvement in blood circulation to the brain stem, which in turn improves the function of the ventral branch of the vagus nerve.

You will probably want to repeat the exercise if necessary.

BASIC OPERATING INSTRUCTIONS

The first few times you train, you should lie on your back. Once you are intimate with these exercises, you can do it sitting in a chair, standing or lying on your back.

1. Lying comfortably on your back, interlace the fingers of one hand with the fingers of the other.

2. Place the hands behind the back of the head, with the weight of the head resting comfortably on the intertwined fingers. You should feel the hardness of the skull with your fingers and you should feel the finger bones on the back of the head. If you have a rigid shoulder and cannot lift both hands behind the back of the head, simply use one hand, with the fingers and the palm in contact with both sides of the back of the head.

3. Holding your head in position, look to the right, moving only your eyes, as far as you can. Don't turn your head; just move your eyes. Keep looking to the right.

 4. After a short period of time, up to thirty or even sixty seconds, you will yawn swallow, or sigh. This is a signal of relaxation in your autonomic nervous system. (A normal inhalation is followed by an exhalation, but a sigh is different; after inhalation, a second inhalation follows the first, before exhalation).

5. Move your eyes again to look straight ahead.

6. Leave your hands in place and make sure you keep your head still. This time, move your eyes to the left.

7. Keep your eyes there until you notice a sigh, a yawn or a swallow.

Now that you've done it, you've completed the basic exercise; remove your hands and sit or stand up.

Evaluate what you've experienced. Has there been any improvement in neck mobility? Has your breath changed? Do you notice anything else?

WHY DO WE MOVE OUR EYES IN THE BASIC EXERCISE?

The basic exercise involves eye movement because there is a direct neurological connection between the eight suboccipital muscles and the muscles that move our eyeballs.

We can directly experience this connection between the movement of the eyes and the changes in the tension of the suboccipital muscles if we place a finger on the back of the head, just below and parallel to the lower edge of the skull. If we leave the head in position, if we move the eyes to the right or left, up or down or diagonally, a slight pressure of the fingers should detect a slight movement of the upper cervical vertebrae or a change in tension levels in the neck muscles below the finger together with every movement of our eyes.

It is noted that socially involved people have a well-positioned C1 and C2. They also have an autonomous nervous system that works well, is flexible and can respond adequately to a variety of situations and internal states.

Social commitment is not a fixed state, nor should the position of C1 and C2 remain fixed after doing the basic exercise. These bones move when our psychological state changes in moments of happiness, satisfaction, fear, anger or abstinence, or when our physiological state changes between social commitment, activation of the dorsal vagus or activation of the spinal sympathetic chain.

Our autonomic nervous system constantly monitors our internal and external environments. When all is well, C1 and C2 enter their place and we get adequate blood flow to the brainstem. When there is a state or vagal dorsal activity of the spinal sympathetic chain, C1 and C2 rotate out of position, reducing blood flow towards the origin of the five cranial nerves in the brain stem and in some areas of the brain. This physiological mechanism takes us away from social commitment, but it also allows us to react when we are challenged or in danger. This mechanism is instinctive, immediate and avoids conscious thought. Usually, we are not aware of the change.

One of the cornerstones of my treatment for stress and depression is realignment of C1 and C2 using the basic exercise or with a practical myofascial release technique. These interventions release imbalances in the tension of the small muscles that support the skull and the first two vertebrae with respect to one another, and this repositions the atlas and the occiput. The better alignment of the vertebrae, in particular C1 and C2, improves blood flow to the brain and generally leads to a rapid improvement in the function of the five nerves necessary for the state of social commitment.

There are other forms of manual therapy that use high and short push speed manipulation techniques designed to implement C1. However, I prefer to use a delicate technique. If I can give the body the right information with a soft touch in the right place, the body will balance itself. Since we cannot implement C1 and C2 and expect them to remain permanently that way, we must repeat the balancing techniques frequently or when necessary. Since there is no state of fixed equilibrium, it is more useful to think of equilibrium as a continuous process.

THE NEUROFASCIAL LIBERATION TECHNIQUE

The basic exercise is a simple self-help method and an easy and effective way to get better function of the ventral vagus nerve. However, if you are a physiotherapist, you may prefer to use your hands instead of exercising people; or you can combine self-help exercises with practical techniques.

The neurofascial release technique can serve as an alternative to the basic exercise. It is particularly useful for treating infants, children and adults on the autistic spectrum who do not have the verbal communication skills needed to absorb the basic exercise instructions, when it can be difficult to communicate with them and have them follow your instructions. Using your hands in this way gives you a nonverbal method to get beneficial changes in another person's nervous system.

If you practice massage or other practical modalities, I suggest you do this technique or that your client does the basic exercise when you start your sessions. This recommendation is in line with the research of Porges, Cottingham and Lyon and will guarantee the flexibility of the client's autonomic nervous system and the maximum benefit from the treatment.

If you are used to massaging, you will have to use your hands in a new way to succeed with this technique. Practice this technique on yourself and learn how to get a release before trying it on another person. To achieve social commitment with this technique, it is necessary to stimulate the reflexes in the nerves of the loose connective tissue just below the skin at the base of the skull. This balances the tension levels in the small muscles between the base of the skull and the vertebrae of the neck.

It will be easier to learn this technique if the person is lying on his stomach, so that you can easily see your fingers. Start with one side of the back of the head.

1. Gently push the base of the skull to one side and feel the hardness of the occipital bone. Test the "sliding ability" of the skin on one side of the occiput. Gently slide the skin over the bone to the right. Then let it go back to neutral.

2. Then slide the skin to the left and let it return to neutral. In which direction was there more resistance?

3. Slide the skin in the direction of maximum resistance. Proceed very slowly and prepare to stop at the first sign of resistance. You may have moved only an eighth of an inch or less. Stop there and keep that position. Continue to feel slight resistance. As you hold that position, the person will sigh or swallow and the resistance in the skin will melt when released.

4. When you perform the test again, the skin should slide easily in both directions.

5. Repeat the technique on the other side.

When evaluating the vagus nerve, it should work properly. Furthermore, there should be greater freedom of movement when turning the head left and right.

INSTRUCTIONS FOR THE TWO-HAND NEUROFASCIAL LIBERATION TECHNIQUE

Once you've trained with one hand, you can use two hands.

1. Place a finger of one hand in the occiput at the base of the back of the head on one side. Test the sliding capacity of the skin on the bone, as described above. The skin should slide more easily in one direction than the other on the bone.

2. Place one finger of the other hand on top of the neck on the same side. If you push a little more, you should be able to feel the muscles. Use this finger to test the ability to slide the skin on the upper neck muscles. It should move more easily in the opposite direction from the direction in which the other finger slides over the skull bone.

3. After the test, relieve the pressure. Let the fingers of your two hands slide the skin in opposite directions until you feel resistance.

4. Stop there and keep that slight tension; wait to sigh or swallow.

5. Release the fingers and allow the skin to return to its original position.

6. Do the same on the skin on the opposite side of the skull and neck.

When you perform the vagus nerve test again, it should now work properly. There should also be greater freedom of movement when turning the head left and right.

APPROPRIATE APPLICATION OF THE NEUROFASCIAL LIBERATION TECHNIQUE

The key to success with the neurofascial release technique is to slide the skin and stop at the first sign of resistance. Use your fingertips to connect with the skin with the lightest touch you can imagine. Then slide the skin a short distance over the underlying layers of muscles, bones and tendons.

This technique differs from the techniques used in other forms of massage, which mainly affect the muscular system and, therefore, push the body. Mainly aim at the muscular system and, therefore, push towards the body. Take the time to read the detailed instructions so you can learn how to do it properly.

This practical technique lengthens the loose connective tissue just under the skin. (To appreciate how fine and delicate this fabric is, go to YouTube and search for "Walking under the skin"). This connective tissue is rich in proprioceptive nerve endings. When you gently slide the skin a very short distance from the muscles and bones, it creates a slight pull in this loose tissue, which is enough to stimulate these nerves.

Slide the skin only a short distance, until you feel the first sign of resistance and, since you are working directly on the proprioceptive nerves, it is not necessary to use the force required by most forms of massage that focus on the muscles. If you use unnecessary force and continue to press after the first sign of resistance, or if you slide the skin too quickly, the muscles and ligaments shrink. It cannot cause any damage in this way: liberation just takes longer. In the worst case, you may not get the changes you want.

You may find that sometimes you are pressing so lightly that the other person reports that they can't feel anything. This is a good response!

As you proceed with the treatment, you will notice an obvious improvement in the skin's ability to slip.

SALAMANDER EXERCISES

The following "salamander exercises" progressively increase the flexibility of the thoracic spine, freeing up the movement of the joints between the individual ribs and the sternum. This will increase the respiratory capacity, help reduce head-forward posture, realign the head again and reduce scoliosis (abnormal spinal curvature).

Eighty percent of the nerve fibers in the vagus are afferent (sensory) fibers, which means that they carry information from the body to the brain, while only 20 percent are efferent (motor) fibers that carry instructions from the brain to the body. Some of the afferent fibers of parts of CN IX and CN X control the amount of oxygen and carbon dioxide in the blood. By improving our breathing pattern with these exercises, we tell the brain (through the afferent nerves) that we are safe and that our visceral organs function properly. This in turn facilitates ventral vagal activity.

But what comes first? Is a limited respiratory pattern the result of a vagal ventral dysfunction or is the lack of function of the ventral vagus caused by the feedback of a non-optimal respiratory pattern? If there are tensions in the respiratory diaphragm and in the muscles that move the ribs, the feedback of the afferent vagal nerves that monitor these movements will signal abnormal breathing, which can prevent a state of ventral vagal activity, in addition to restoring the activity of the ventral vagus improving physiological conditions; in practice, improving both is useful, regardless of which one came first.

A head-forward posture reduces the space in the upper part of the chest that is available for breathing. Salamander exercises can create more space in the upper chest for the heart and lungs. Reducing head-forward posture will also eliminate pressure on nerves ranging from the spinal cord to the heart, lungs and visceral organs. By improving the alignment of the cervical vertebrae, the salamander exercises also relieve the pressure on the vertebral arteries and can relieve some back pain between the shoulders.

When you perform the salamander exercises, bring your head to the same level as the rest of the spinal column. This posture is similar to that of a salamander, which has no neck, so its head is like an extra vertebra in the upper part of the spine. A salamander cannot flex, extend, rotate or bend the head separately from the first vertebra of the spine, nor lift the head above the level of the vertebrae as well as reptiles and mammals.

This exercise is performed with the head aligned with the spine. The thoracic part (part of the thorax of the spine) can now bend better, like a salamander. You can use lateral flexing movements in the thoracic vertebrae to loosen muscle tension between the ribs and the thoracic spine. This contributes to the freedom of movement of the ribs and promotes optimal breathing.

In the extension and flexion of the human spine, there is usually greater flexibility in the neck and lumbar vertebrae and less flexibility in the thoracic spine. However, the flexibility of the thoracic spine increases considerably with lateral flexion. The facet joints of the thoracic vertebrae are unlocked, which allows the thoracic spine to bend more freely.

THE MIDDLE SALAMANDER: A VARIATION

In this variation of the half salamander exercise, follow the same instructions above, but let your eyes look to the right while tilting your head to the left (figure 11). This movement of your eyes in the opposite direction before moving your head increases your range of motion; you should be able to tilt your head to one side, hold this for thirty to sixty seconds, and then do the same on the other side.

LEVEL 2: THE FULL SALAMANDER EXERCISE

The complete salamander exercise involves the lateral rotation of the entire vertebral column rather than just the neck. Furthermore, we use a different body position.

1. Get on all fours, supporting your weight on your knees and palms. You can put your hands on the floor, but it's better if you put your palms on a table, a chair seat or a sofa cushion. Your head should be on the same level as the spine

2. In this exercise, the ears should not rise or fall below the level of the spine. To find the correct position of the head, slightly raise your head over what you think is correct. You should be able to feel that your head is slightly raised. Then lower your head slightly below what you think is right. You should be able to feel that your head is lower than it should be. Come and go between the two positions. Raise your head a little mnd then lower it a little. Try to find a position in the middle where the head does not sit too high or low. Although

you may never find this exact position, you can start focusing on it.

3. After finding a good position for the head in relation to the spine, look to the right with the eyes, hold them in that position and bend the head to the right, moving the right ear towards the right shoulder.

4. Complete the movement by letting the curve of your side continue beyond the neck to the base of the spine.

5. Hold this position for thirty or sixty seconds.

6. Bring the spine and head back to the center.

7. Repeat all the previous steps, but on the left side.

SCM EXERCISE FOR STIFF NECK

This exercise extends your range of motion as you turn your head, relieves stiff neck symptoms and helps prevent migraines. It is similar to the first movements we made when we were children lying on our stomachs, leaning on our elbows, our heads free to move so we could look around.

1. Lie down on your stomach. Raise your head and put your arms under your chest. Support the weight of the upper body on the elbows.

2. Turn your head to the right side as far as you can go. Hold that position for sixty seconds.

3. Bring your head to the center.

4. Now turn your head to the left as far as possible and keep that position for sixty seconds.

If the rotation of the head has improved with this exercise, but the movement is still not as good as you would like it to be on one side, then the restriction probably comes from another muscle, the elevated scapula, which is innervated by the spinal nerves C3 – C5. This type of torticollis will not be eliminated only by improving the function of CN XI and the trapezius and sternocleidomastoid muscles.

Part of the stiffness may also come from a hiatal hernia and shortening of the esophagus, as the vagus nerve is wrapped around the esophagus.

TWIST AND TURN EXERCISE FOR THE TRAPEZIUS

The twist and turn exercise improves the tone of a flaccid trapezius muscle and balances each of its three parts with the other two parts. It also helps to stretch the spine, improve breathing and correct head-forward posture (FHP). This in turn relieves shoulder and back pain.

This exercise can be of benefit to anyone, not just those with FHP. It takes less than a minute to do it and the feeling of positive change is immediate. It is a good idea that you take a moment to do this exercise when you've been sitting for a while and repeat it regularly from time to time. I do it almost every time I get up from sitting at my computer. Each time you train, you will experience improved breathing and posture and its positive effects are cumulative.

The belief behind this exercise is not to strengthen or lengthen the trapezius muscle. The assumption is that the muscle is strong enough and only needs nerve stimulation for flaccid muscle fibers. It is waking them up so they can take care of their part of the job, like they did when we were kids and crawled on all fours.

When a child lies on his stomach, he uses all the fibers of the three parts of the trapezius muscle to hold the shoulder blades together, lift the head and turn the head to look around. Later, the child also uses all these muscle fibers when he gets on all fours to look around.

However, when a child stands up, all the trapezius fibers are no longer used evenly. Some become more tense, while energy leaves other fibers to become flabby. The three parts of the trapezius muscle no longer hold the head in the same way. Over time, the head tends to slide further forward, so that the centers of the ears are in front of the center of the shoulders. The shoulders show a tendency to pull forward and down towards the midline.

After doing this exercise, you will have a more uniform tone in all the muscle fibers of the three parts of your trapezius. So, when you stand up or sit down, your head will slide back and forth naturally, reducing FHP and improving your posture.

INSTRUCTIONS FOR THE TWIST AND TURN EXERCISE

There are three parts to this exercise. The difference between the three parts is the position of the arms.

1. Sit comfortably on a solid surface, such as a chair or a bench. Keep your face neutral.

2. Fold and cross your arms, with your hands resting lightly on your elbows. You will quickly turn the shoulder girdle, first on one side and then on the other, without stopping and without moving your hips.

3. For the first part of the exercise, drop your elbows and rest in front of your body. Rotate the shoulders so that the elbows move, first to one side and then to the other. When you turn your shoulders from side to side, your arms slide slightly on your stomach. This activates the fibers of the upper trapezius.

4. Do it three times. Do not strain yourself or stop your movements. Move your shoulders without forcing or holding them; your movements should be easy and relaxed.

5. The second part is the same as the first; the only difference is that you raise your elbows and keep them in front of your chest, at the level of your heart. Rotate your elbows first to one side and then to the other. Do it three times. This activates the muscle fibers of your middle trapezius.

6. For the third part, raise your elbows as high as you can and repeat the previous exercise. Rotate your elbows from side to side three times. This activates the muscle fibers of the lower trapezius.

After training, you may notice that your head feels lighter and has moved back and forth, away from the head-forward position. It is not uncommon for someone with a significant

FHP to be more than an inch or two taller after the first time you train. If someone looks at you from one side, they will see that your head has moved a little back from its original position forward, if you've had that trend.

A FOUR-MINUTE NATURAL FACE LIFT, PART 1

The benefits of this gentle and pleasant treatment include relaxation of the facial muscles and a more natural smile by improving the function of the cranial nerves V and VII. You can do it yourself and share it with others.

This exercise:

- Improves circulation in the skin.
- It gives life to the muscles of expression of the middle third of the face, in the area between the corners of the mouth and the corners of the eyes.
- It improves blood circulation in the skin of the face.
- Provides a youthful quality of liveliness that you can feel and that others can see.
- Helps you smile more naturally and more frequently.
- Makes your face respond better to interactions with others and therefore increases your sense of empathy.
- Makes the cheekbones more prominent and the cheeks very high a little flatter.

Before doing this technique, look at your face in a mirror. If you are doing the technique with another person, hold a hand mirror so you can look at your face and follow the changes. Look in particular at the area of the skin around the cheekbones.

Do one side of the face first. Check if you can see or hear a difference between the two sides. The differences are generally evident when you talk or smile. Then do the other side. There should be more symmetry again.

WHERE TO DO THE TECHNIQUE

There is a point on the face which is the end point of the acupuncture meridian of the large intestine, called LI 20. It is a point of beauty in Chinese, Japanese and Thai massage. In classic Thai massage, this point is called "Golden Bamboo". In traditional Chinese medicine, this point is called "welcome fragrance" and opens the nostrils, improving breathing.

This point in Chinese medicine is interesting in terms of Western anatomy. It is located directly on a joint between two facial bones, the jaw and the premaxilla. The two bones were separate entities long ago in the evolutionary development of our species, but they were calcified together in a single bone at an early stage. In modern anatomy, the maxilla/premaxilla is known as a bone called the jaw.

The end point of the large intestine meridian is easy to find. Just lightly touch the skin about an eighth of an inch from the top of the above-the-wing fold (the fold between the cheek and the upper lip), near the outer edge of the nose. If you explore the area with a finger, you will find this point easily because it is more sensitive than the rest of the surrounding skin.

HOW AND WHY OF THE TECHNIQUE

The surface of the skin of the face is innervated by the branches of the fifth cranial nerve. Lightly touching the skin of the face stimulates these nerve endings.

1. With very light contact, brush the surface of the skin at the LI 20 acupuncture point. Then let the fingertip melt together with the skin.

2. Slide the skin up and down to find which way has more resistance. Push lightly on that resistance.

3. Hold at that point and wait for the release.

4. Slide the skin inward, towards the midline of the face and toward the side to find the direction of maximum resistance.

5. Stop there and push slightly. Wait for the release.

The muscles of the face are innervated by the branches of the seventh cranial nerve (VII). There are two layers of facial muscles just below the skin.

6. Let the tip of your finger gently sink into the muscle layers under the skin at the same point. Let the first muscular layer adhere to the tip of the finger as if it were Velcro.

7. If you are careful not to press too hard and if you feel what is happening under your fingers, you can slide these layers of

muscles. First slide one layer over the other, forming a small circle.

8. As you move around the circle, you may notice greater resistance in one direction. Continue to press lightly in that direction and hold it until it is released in the form of a sigh or swallow.

9. Then, push a little deeper. Now the deeper layer of muscles join the upper muscular layer and the skin. You can slide both layers together on the bone surface.

10. As you move around the circle, you may notice greater resistance in one direction. Continue to press lightly in that direction and hold it until it is released in the form of a sigh or swallow.

All bones have a covering of connective tissue called periosteum (peri means "around" and osteo means "bone"). This tissue is very rich in nerve endings of the spinal nerves or, in this case, of the cranial nerves.

11. Let the tip of your finger sink deeper into your face until it rests lightly on the surface of the bone.

12. Massage on the periosteum surface has a profound effect on the autonomic nervous system. Press lightly, but hard enough to reach the surface of the bone in the large intestine 20. Let the fingertips move from side to side on the surface of the bone. Keep light pressure on the bone and wait for it to be free.

In the embryo, this was two bones, the jaw and the premaxilla. Although these have merged into a single bone, it is still possible to feel that once there were two separate bones.

This massage to cranial nerves V and VII stimulates the skin's nerves and facial muscles. It does not erase all wrinkles, but relaxes the muscles of the face, reduces some wrinkles and leaves the face younger and fresher. And there are no negative side effects like scar tissue from a lifting operation or toxic accumulations of Botox.

More importantly, this massage helps the face to be more expressive, communicative and receptive, more socially engaged. Our face must be flexible and able to express different emotional responses in various situations. Facial expressions are a vital part of our communication with other people.

In addition to expressing our emotions, face flexibility is important for social commitment. When our face is relaxed and we look at another person's face, our own face automatically performs micro-movements that reflect the other's facial expression. These movements are very small and change very quickly.

These changes of tension in our skin and in our facial muscles feed the brain, through the afferent pathways of cranial nerves V and VII, to give us immediate information on the subconscious feelings of others. This is a prerequisite for us to feel empathy for another person.

If the facial muscles under the skin are generally relaxed, a person usually has a soft and pleasant face and one that looks beautiful or handsome.

Unfortunately, many people remain trapped in the same emotional and facial pattern for years. The facial muscles pull the skin, creating wrinkles or a double chin. If the person remains in the same emotional state and does not relax the facial muscles, these wrinkles deepen over time.

In addition to this technique, a slight movement of the facial skin stimulates the CN V and reduces tension in all facial muscles.

A FOUR-MINUTE NATURAL FACE LIFT, PART 2

Part 1 focuses on LI20, an acupuncture point in the large intestine meridian near the nostril. Stimulating this point improves the balance and tone of the muscles of the lower face around the mouth and nose. Part 2, in turn, focuses on the eyes. The real technique is similar in many ways to the first face-stretching technique you did in the large intestine 20. You will find the acupuncture point B2 in the inner corner of the eyebrow. People often rub this point naturally, without thinking, when they are tired. Massaging the skin and facial muscles here is often relaxing.

Using your thumb or finger, connect to B2. In B2, go down each of the layers: the skin, two layers of muscles and the periosteum.

This point is also a trigger point for the eye's orbicular muscle, a thin and flat muscle that surrounds the eye opening. Sometimes the eyes are called the mirror of the soul. Before working on the B2, the muscle could be too tight, leaving the eye a little closed or it could be without a twist, leaving the eye too open. When we finish, there will be a better balance between looking outside and looking inside. You will see another person more clearly, and this person in turn will make eye contact with you easier and you will experience seeing differently.

At a deeper level, this acupuncture point is located on the edge of a small facial bone called the lacrimal bone, often referred to as the tear bone. Sometimes a person's eyes can be dry and appear lifeless. Some might even experience an annoying flow of tears. By touching this bone in B2 and maintaining contact on the tear bone, it will balance the flow of moisture in the eyes and leave them bright and shiny. The aim of the lifting massage is to leave a smile on the lips and a sparkle in the eyes.

1. Find the place in the inner corner of the eyebrow that is more sensitive than the surrounding areas.

2. First, use your finger to lightly brush the skin.

3. Leave the tip of your finger resting lightly on the skin at point B2 (see above) and maintain that contact with the surface of the skin until it is released as a sigh or swallow.

4. Then, gently press down on the muscular layer of the face. This is where the flat and round orbicular muscle that

surrounds the eye adheres to the bones of the face. Let the skin stick to your finger and form a small circle, making the skin slip slightly and looking for the direction in which there is resistance.

5. Keep your finger on that resistance until it is released as a sigh or swallow.

6. Then go even deeper until you feel the surface of the bone. Rub it a couple of times.

7. Then maintain contact with the bone and wait for release.

If the orbicularis muscle of the eyelids is too narrow, closing the eyelids and narrowing the eyes, this should open the eye more normally. If the eye was too open, this technique should reaffirm it a little but leave it open.

IN SUMMARY

The purpose of all these self-help exercises and practical techniques is to help people get out of a vagal dorsal state, or to help them get out of the chronic activation of the sympathetic chain, and to bring them home in a ventral vagal state. Only then can we cut off all the heads of the Hydra and restore our capacity for physical and emotional health.

CONCLUSION

WAYS TO UNLOCK THE
VAGUS NERVE'S POWERS

IMPULSE WITH ELECTRICITY

Doctors have used the nerve's influence in the brain for a long time. Electrical stimulation of the vagus nerve is most times used to treat people with epilepsy or depression. By sending regular pulses of electricity to the brain through the vagus nerve, VNS is designed to prevent seizures. A device similar to a pacemaker provides these pulses. It is placed in the chest wall under the skin and a cord runs from it to the neck's vagus nerve. Studies investigating the effects of ambiguous stimulation on epilepsy noticed that patients had a second advantage unrelated to seizure reduction: their mood also improved.

TECHNIQUES FOR VAGUS NERVE STIMULATION

The vagus nerve need not be in shape. In a similar way to a muscle, it can also tone and strengthen. Here are a few simple things you can do that will improve your health significantly:

1. Positive social relationships: A study led the participants to think about others with empathy, silently repeating optimistic sentences about friends and family. The meditators showed a

general increase in positive emotions like serenity, joy and hope after the lesson was completed compared to the controls. These other positive thoughts have contributed to an increase in vagal function as seen in variation in heart rate. The results also revealed a more tonic vagus nerve than simple meditation.

2. Cold: "It also activates the nerve by exposure to cold, like cold showers or immersion in the head."

Studies show that when your body adapts to the cold, your (sympathetic nerve) combat or flight system decreases and your (parasympathetic) rest and digestion system increases, and the vagus nerve mediates this. Every form of acute cold exposure, including drinking ice water, may increase activation of the vagus nerve.

3. Gargle: Another home remedy is to gargle with water for a vagus nerve with little stimulation. Gargling directly stimulates the muscles of the palette that the vagus nerve stimulates.

"Patients usually break up a little, which is a good sign, and if not, we suggest doing it every day until they know they start crying a little," Hoffman says. "This has been shown to instantly improve the performance of working memory."

4. Singing and humming: Humming, prayer chanting, hymn singing, and positive and enthusiastic chanting increase heart rate variability (HRV) in slightly different ways. Singing is essentially like beginning a vagal bomb that sends waves of relaxation. The singing in the upper part of the lungs serves to activate the vagus on the back muscles of the throat.

Singing alone, often performed in churches and synagogues, also increases HRV and vagal function. Singing has been found to boost oxytocin, also known as the love hormone because it makes people feel good and closer to each other.

5. Massage: The vagus nerve can be aroused by massaging the feet and neck along the carotid sinus situated on either side of the neck along the carotid arteries. A massage of the neck may help to reduce seizures. A foot massage help can reduce blood pressure and heart rate. The vagus nerve can also be keyed up by a pressure massage. Such massages are used in enhancing bowel function to help children gain weight, mainly induced by vagus nerve stimulation.

6. Laughter: Happiness and laughter are natural immune enhancers. Laughter stimulates the vagus nerve as well. Research shows that laughter in a group environment raises the HRV.

There are a lot of cases of people who have laughing faints, and this may be due to the parasympathetic process of the vagus nerve being too stimulated. In addition to urinating, coughing, swallowing or defecating, fainting can occur after laughter, which is favored by the activation of the vagus nerve.

7. Yoga and tai chi: Both improve vagus nerve function and generally increase the parasympathetic system. Studies have shown that GABA, a relaxing neurotransmitter in the brain, is enhanced by yoga. Researchers believe it "stimulates vagal afferents (fibers)," which enhances the function of the

parasympathetic nervous system. This is particularly helpful for those that are suffering from anxiety or depression. Studies show that tai chi can "enhance vagal modulation" as well.

8. Deep and steady breathing: Neurons in the heart and neck called baroreceptors sense blood pressure and relay the neuronal signal to the brain. They stimulate the heart-connecting vagus nerve to reduce blood pressure and heart rate. Slow breathing increases the sensitivity of the baroreceptors and vagal activation with approximately the same amount for inhalation and exhalation. It can be very beneficial to take around 5-6 breaths per minute in an average adult.

9. Exercise: Exercise increases the hormone of brain growth, protects the mitochondria of the brain and helps to reverse cognitive impairment. Yet stimulating the vagus nerve has also been shown, resulting in beneficial effects on cognitive and brain health. Smooth physical exercise also stimulates the vagus nerve-mediated intestinal flow.

10. Coffee enemas: That's right, enemas for the vagus nerve are like sprints. The expansion of the stomach, as is the case for enemas, increases the activation of the vagus nerve. Such cleaning is achieved by increasing the capacity of the liver to detoxify and bind to bile blood toxins. By releasing toxic bile into the small intestine and then into the large intestine for evacuation, the liver is drained. Every three minutes all the blood supply circulates through the liver. The blood will circulate about four to five times for cleaning, as well as a

dialysis treatment, by storing the coffee for 12-15 minutes. The content of coffee water stimulates intestinal peristalsis and helps with accumulated toxic bile to empty the large intestine.

11. Nervana: This portable drug sends a gentle electrical pulse through the left ear canal to activate the body's vagus nerve, synchronizing with the beat, which in effect induces the release of neurotransmitters in the brain to create a relaxing sensation.

12 Throughout the entire body: Relax: The most important thing to help keep the vagus nerve toned can be to learn to relax. Many calming practices, according to Hoffman, will activate the vagus nerve.